THE
ENOUGHNESS
Method

RECLAIMING YOUR POWER, WORTH & PEACE AFTER BURNOUT

CARRIE
SEVERSON

The Enoughness Method

Published in the United States by the Unapologetic Voice House. The Unapologetic Voice House is a hybrid publishing house focused on publishing strong female voices and stories.

www.theunapologeticvoicehouse.com

The Enoughness Method is the result of years of research and personal experience.

ISBN: 978-1-955090-32-2 (Paperback) 978-1-955090-33-9 (E-Book)

Library of Congress Control Number: 2023948170

To Gavin:
What a ride, right?
I love you.
Unapologetically.

CONTENTS

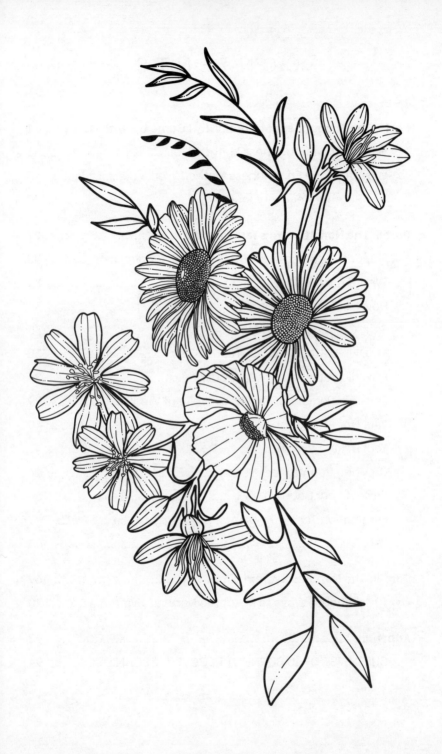

PART I

The Enoughness Method: Why I Came Up with It

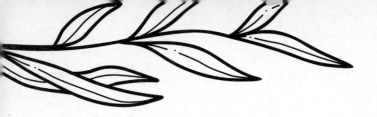

I NEVER HEARD the term "burnout" prior to waking up on my 35th birthday. My eyes popped open, and it was the first thing that ran through my mind.

Burnout.

I grabbed my phone from inside the nightstand drawer and tapped the internet icon. I typed the word "burnout" into a search field and waited.

I read the first definition I saw.

Burnout: a state of emotional, mental, or physical exhaustion caused from excessive prolonged stress.

A dam of tears broke free from my eye sockets.

Finally.

Finally, I had a word to describe what I was experiencing.

Burnout.

That was it. I was burned out. After months of fatigue, weight gain, sleepless nights, diminished interest in my work, and disconnection from my personal life, I could slap a word on it.

I couldn't breathe for a few seconds. A panic attack surged through my body. I put one hand on my heart and the other on my belly, focusing on getting air in and out. I was used to panic attacks. I didn't try to hold back the tears. Ugly, *ugly* crying, deep, ugly crying.

I let the panic run its course and focused on my breathing as tears rolled down my cheeks.

I am safe.

I am safe.

I am safe.

I sat up and looked at myself in the mirror across the room. I ran my hands softly over my cheeks and down my neck, drying the tears with the palms of my hands.

For several months leading up to that day, I saw a naturopath on a regular basis. She had me on different homeopathic medications for anxiety, stress, resentment, guilt, embarrassment, and shame. Her goal was to help me address these issues, though we never actually talked about my health in that dire state. My mental health was fragile though. I was bone tired and on a roller coaster of emotions every day.

That day was a breaking point for me. Knowing what was going on was the first step. Accepting myself as a burnout was the second step. Figuring out what to do about it was the third step.

In 2013, very few people were talking about burnout. It wasn't widely discussed—at least it wasn't known in my circles of entrepreneurs, leaders, and young professionals. It wasn't like I could sit down at a luncheon or dinner and ask women at the table about their experience with it.

I burned out because I was unprepared for my own success. Years prior, I created an organization from the ground up. It was called Severson Sisters. It was a bullying solutions organization for young girls. I launched it in 2011, and it took off running weeks after I hit the go button. So did I:

Speaking gigs.

Media segments.

Fundraisers.

Published books.

An afterschool program.

Managing boards and volunteers.

I didn't stop until that morning in 2013. The morning I heard the term *burnout* for the first time was the day I surrendered.

And that wasn't easy.

As a born entrepreneur and trailblazer, surrendering felt like failure at first. I didn't want to surrender because giving up my hustle, my warrior badge, the armor, and my burnout made me question my own success.

Was I successful if I couldn't keep up with the demand and handle everything?

That morning I made a deal with myself.

As I ran my hands over my protruding breasts and down my body that I didn't recognize anymore because of the fifty additional pounds I absorbed over the years, I called myself a burnout, and agreed to give myself a year to recover.

I agreed to let myself recover without the super loud, critical voice who also questioned whether or not I was a successful entrepreneur, a disruptor, trailblazer, influencer, and a positive changemaker because I was also a

burnout. I told her to take a nap and let the big piece of me that had been neglected for years come out to shine.

I took a year to play, and the more life I allowed to happen for me, the better I felt.

I went down a rabbit hole and researched burnout daily, searching for answers. It wasn't a new concept, coined in the mid-1970s by a man named Herbert Freudenberger.

The deeper down the bunny hole I went, the more frustrated I became because recovery advice stopped after time-management tips, mid-day power naps, breathing exercises, and getting more sunshine and fresh air.

I wasn't surprised there wasn't a road to recovery already laid out for me to follow. I figured, though, I was an entrepreneur and running a nonprofit by myself, so I could carve out a recovery path for myself. I was confident I could trailblaze my way out of the burnout hole I had fallen into.

As I recovered from burnout, I shared my experience with people through my writing, on stage through personal storytelling, and in person. I shared things that helped me move out of burnout, such as getting outside for exercise, taking deeper breaths, cuddling with the dog, and putting boundaries around my time so I could meditate more and stress less. I shared how I found happiness and peace within myself again, along with self-care tools and nervous system recalculating maneuvers.

People responded by telling me about their own experience with extreme fatigue, feelings of everything, including themselves, being lackluster, and even tips from their therapists, friends, and priests.

Everyone had a different approach to burnout recovery. However, the common thread amongst us was that we wanted to feel alive again.

At some point in my journey, a light bulb went off above my head. Actually, it was more like a big flashing neon sign.

It said... *Write a book...write a book...write a book.* I call those big flashing signs a few different things:

Spidey. My sixth sense. God. The Universe. Women's intuition.

The big flashing signs always stopped me in my tracks, took my breath away, scared the bejesus out of me, and typically got a verbal or written response from me. Sometimes my responses included cuss words.

That particular sign got a written response.

Hey God.

Seriously? You want me to write a book now? That's a lot of work. How do I fill a book with this? What should I say? I don't want to write a book about burnout. I'm still managing burnout after doing the last thing you told me to do. I don't want to do this.

I love you despite this new task you're asking me to do, but no way.

Love,

Carrie

Whenever signs showed up from the Universe I either disagreed with or got scared by, this overwhelming tug-of-war between my heart, head, and gut took place. My coach called the tug-of-war, plain 'ol resistance. It was true.

Writing a book about my burnout in 2013 and my recovery since was something I was scared to do. I was scared because of the amount of work I knew it would require, and I was scared of burning out again.

I had hundreds upon hundreds of emails from readers of my published pieces on the *Huffington Post* about my burnout journey. I didn't disagree with the need for a book about burnout, but....

My brain kept me from taking one more leap of faith I was asked to do. My inner dialogue was screaming crap, like...

What if you burnout again?

This is going to be hard work.

How are you going to make money doing this?

All those things were big rocks. There were not any pebble-size thoughts floating around inside my head. Writing a book is hard work. And it's intense and can easily be isolating, stressful, and emotionally draining. By that time in my life, I had been through writing books a few times, but I didn't have a clear direction on how to write about my burnout journey.

I took some time with this new request from God. I journaled about it. After months and months of procrastination, I came back to the same answer over and over again.

In my thirty-five years on the planet, the biggest life lesson I received came down to a simple statement: My intuition is my superpower, and it is always right.

Always.

I knew that when I ignored big flashing neon signs from God, my life got harder. It was always better to listen to my intuition. To God. To spidey. To the Universe.

So I started writing a book. I immersed myself in the world of writing. I went to conferences, worked on expanding my platform, and wrote personal essays about my life for national magazines. I spent months writing a book proposal and created a list of 100 literary agents I would have loved to work with on my book.

As I pitched, the Universe gave me signs that I was going in the right direction.

One afternoon, in New York City, I felt the urge to leave a conference I was attending and get out in the sunshine and just walk. I walked and walked until I saw this one spot of sunlight on a monument in Columbus Circle. I knew I was meant to sit in that one spot and take a deep breath and wait. After a few minutes of enjoying the sun on my face I noticed a woman staring at me.

"Can I help you?" I asked.

"I'm sitting here trying to figure out how not to burn out at my job," she said right back to me.

"Oh well, I can help you there. I'm recovering from burnout. What do you do for a living?"

"I'm a literary agent," she said.

I didn't say anything back for a few beats. Chills ran up and down my body. The hair on the back of my neck stood up, and angel bumps covered my arms and legs. I shared self-care techniques that really helped me—fresh air, closing my eyes and box breathing, or sticking my face in cold water. Eventually, I told her about my book and asked if I could send it to her. She agreed, and I heard back from her a month later.

She loved it. She related to it. She cried. She laughed. And it killed her to pass on it. She was the first literary agent to say that my book was as good as books on the *New York Times* best-seller lists, but because I didn't have a platform, she couldn't sell it.

Because I didn't have a big enough platform, the book wasn't sellable.

I pitched agent after agent after that first rejection. I was compared to literary giants for years and always rejected. It was heartbreaking and hard to see a response from an agent and in their email read names of big-time authors I admired and adored. I wasn't told that my product wasn't good enough. In fact, it was the opposite.

The issue was, *I wasn't enough for agents.* My work, my platform, my voice weren't enough for them. I kept going and stayed persistent. In the end, I pitched to nearly 100 agents. I firmly believed I was meant to deliver this book about burnout to other burnouts in the world.

Despite refusing to give up, I questioned what I was doing and why I was doing it.

Am I doing this for fame?

Am I doing this to get rich?

How am I going to compete with those women who have big names, big budgets, and famous friends?

The truth was, I wasn't. I wasn't doing any of it: able to compete or trying to get a traditional book deal for fame or for riches. I knew that. There was a strong drive guiding me forward. I was meant to get this book about burnout and burnout recovery out.

When I met Gavin, the man I would one day call my husband, in 2018, I put it down for a little while. I loved being in a new relationship. Everything was fresh and unknown. Every touch sent thrills through my body. But in the fall of that year, my next message from the Universe jolted me awake. I was lying in bed next to Gavin when it happened.

Be the house.

It was a message I felt echoing deep down throughout my whole body. My heart ached. My stomach dropped. And just like it had happened on my 35th birthday when I heard the word *burnout* for the first time, my eyes were barely open for the day when it happened.

Be the house.

This time, I jumped out of bed, shaking my finger up to the heavens and screaming out loud.

"F*ck that, God. I am not creating one more thing here. Be the house, no way."

Gavin leapt out of bed and landed in his ready-to-fight stance. Across the bed from me, wild haired, big eyes, knees bent, fists clenched, able to defend us against an intruder, Gavin searched the room for an intruder, because the only reason I'd be screaming first thing in the morning would be because of an intruder.

He blinked at me a few times.

I played it off.

"What are you doing?" I asked, laughing, trying to hide my smile.

"What was that?"

"What's what?"

"I heard something," he said.

"Like what?"

"You screamed."

"What?"

I was going to keep this going until he gave up.

It didn't take long for Gavin to sigh and crawl back into bed. I went downstairs for coffee and meditation on the couch. I didn't want to have a conversation with him about spidey and the new request it gave me for my life direction.

I plopped down in the nook of the couch with my coffee in one hand and a journal and pen in the other. I crossed my legs and exhaled. I set my cup down on the window ledge and cracked the window open to get some fresh air. The scent of my freshly brewed cup of coffee mixed with a brand-new day comforted me. With my eyes closed, I focused on my breathing.

Exhale.

Hold.

Inhale.

Hold.

After a few minutes, I felt centered in my body. I let my mind swirl around the message I received upstairs.

Be the house.

I took a long drag of coffee, grabbed my pen and journal, and wrote a letter to God.

Dear God, I know what you mean. Be the house means you want me to start another business and not just any business. You want me to start a publishing house for people like me—authors who are compared to giants

and passed on because they don't know the right peo-
ple or don't have the right amount of cash or platform
numbers. I don't want to do that. There isn't a singu-
lar cell in my body that wants to create a new business
that actually operates as a publishing house. I am in a
fairly new relationship with Gavin. It's going well. We'll
end up getting married, and I just want to settle into this
new thing in my life. My storytelling coaching business
is going well. Life is really great. I don't want to rock the
boat. I love you.

Carrie

I ignored the message. For months on end, I did what I could to push *Be the house* out of the corner of my mind. And the more I ignored the message, the more my storytelling business dried up. It didn't take long for me to realize what was happening. I couldn't ignore *Be the house* anymore. In early 2019, I gave myself two choices: I could find a full-time job, or I could create a publishing house. One morning, while meditating on the couch, I took a good look inward and asked myself why I resisted creating a new business. I asked myself that question the last time my spidey sense gave me a directive. This time, instead of resisting writing a book, I was resisting creating a publishing house.

The same answers came up.

What if I burnout again?

This is going to be hard work.

How are you going to make money doing this?

Again, all those things were big rocks. No small things swimming around inside my head. I knew all too well the challenges of launching and running a business. Burnout was a real possibility. Running a business, especially a new business, is intense and can easily be as isolating as writing a book. It can be stressful and emotionally draining.

Do I really feel safe launching a new business?

"Can I do this and NOT burnout?" is the real question.

I could feel anxiety rise up in my belly. I was so scared of burning out again, and I hadn't even started. Suddenly, a huge well of unexpected tears sprung from my eyes, and my breath stuck in my chest. I stood up and shook my limbs to get myself out of fight-or-flight mode. I immediately started tapping the side of my palm.

I am safe.

I am safe.

I am safe.

I moved my tapping around my eye socket, down my face, onto my collar bone, under my arm, and on the top of my head. After a few rounds of tapping, I felt calm and got a yawn out.

I sat back down on the couch, opened the window next to me, and sat there for a few minutes with my eyes closed, just focusing on the way the breeze felt on my skin.

After a few minutes, I did my breathing exercise.

Deep breath in, hold it, deep exhale, hold it.

In. Hold. Exhale.

Inhale. Hold. Exhale.

Last time through.

The anxiety subsided but I could still feel the residue of it. I climbed out of the corner of the couch and jumped into the shower quickly, knowing the shock of the cold water would snap me out of it and help me feel grounded, back in my body, and safe again.

That was my real method. I turned to three things most often when I felt my fight-or-flight kick in.

Silence in fresh air.

Box breath.

A cold shower.

It was the method I used to bring me back to one simple fact.

I was enough. As I was.

It was my enoughness method.

What Is the Enoughness Method?

Whenever I felt a surge of anxiety, massively overwhelmed, or couldn't take a deep breath, I found fresh air, box breathing, and a cold shower were the three self-care and nervous system recalculating tools that helped me the most.

Fresh air, box breathing, and a cold shower were so effective for me climbing out of burnout, I named it The Enoughness Method and started timing it. The whole method is over within six minutes, and I went through the method several times a day in the thick of burnout. I'd start my day with The Enoughness Method. I'd do it again before I got ready for bed. And if I needed to do it in the middle of the day, I'd do it then, too.

The Enoughness Method is as simple as 3, 2, 1.

Or, 1, 2, 3

Or any combination of them all!

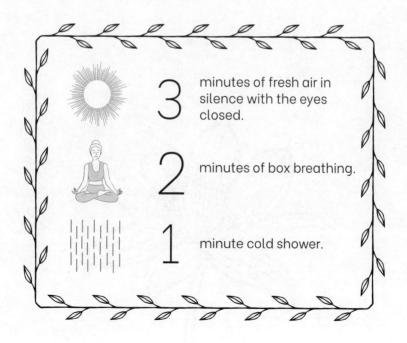

3 minutes of fresh air in silence with the eyes closed.

2 minutes of box breathing.

1 minute cold shower.

Fresh air does a body good. When I was a kid, I was always told to go outside and play. I had recess. We ate meals outside. I played in treehouses and on swing sets. I'd meet friends at parks just to sit on benches.

Fresh air is important to calming down the nervous system. The key is to be present outside. Leave your phone and all the other trinkets and devices inside for three minutes. You'll know when three minutes have passed up. It's just enough time for your body to relax before your mind searches for the next thought to occupy itself. Watch clouds roll by. Look at the trees, leaves, the shape of the windows, bricks, or sidewalk. Just be present with fresh air.

To effectively perform box breathing, you will exhale for four counts, hold your breath for four counts, inhale for four counts and hold again for four counts. Repeat that pattern for two minutes.

And the cold water is a great way to get your body back in harmony. If you don't have access to a shower at all times, splash cold water on your face, or put a cold water bottle on the side of your neck.

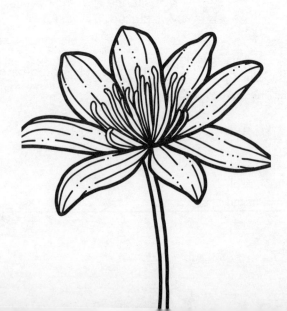

Why Does the Enoughness Method Work?

Burnout isn't something I just fell into. It didn't happen to me, or you for that matter, because we have bad bosses, crazy co-workers, or because we're underpaid and overworked. Granted, none of that helps make life any better, easier, or more fun in any way. But when it's all said and done, burnout happens because of a lack of boundaries, a lack of self-care, self-love, self-compassion, and most importantly not seeing oneself as enough.

In case you don't know if you're burned out though, check your internal dialogue against what the World Health Organization said about it. The WHO defined burnout as an occupational phenomenon in 2019 and called burnout a syndrome resulting from chronic workplace stress that has not been successfully managed.

And let's face it, when we are exposed to long-term unmanaged stress in our daily lives, our mental, emotional, physical, and spiritual selves are frayed.

Mine was.

Burnout happened over the course of years.

It happened because I kept saying yes to things. I worked really long hours, hoping to accomplish something that would bring in more money, more recognition, more support. I took calls at all hours of the day and night, on the weekends, and never spoke up about the number of tasks piled up on my desk, to-do lists, or in notebooks. No matter what I did, it was never enough. I never felt like it was enough or like I was enough.

Burnout is characterized typically by a combination of several symptoms. Exhaustion is the number one reported symptom in burnout studies. Being bone tired was an issue I faced day after day because I never prioritize my own self-tenderness. I worked and worked and worked until I couldn't keep my eyes open anymore. No matter how many hours of sleep I got each night, it didn't help and having four cups of coffee throughout the day was necessary and still pointless.

In addition to physical exhaustion, burnout is also characterized by feelings of cynicism and apathy. For me, cynicism came in strong. So strong it brought me into a state of resentment quickly before landing on the feeling of apathy in the end.

Since COVID, one symptom of burnout was coined quiet quitting. When that term popped up, I thought back to my own actions in 2013. Quiet quitting became known as the state where employees aren't doing anything above and beyond their actual job description. I get it. I worked between set hours, left at a certain time, and didn't work on the weekends. That was necessary for my own recovery.

There are a lot of symptoms for burnout. Depression. Headaches. Sleeplessness. Weight gain. Weight loss. Extreme feelings of being overwhelmed. Brain fog. I had all of it. Except for the weight loss. I'm part Irish, German, and Viking. We come out big and strong.

When apathy set in sometime in 2013, I finally surrendered. There was nowhere else left to go but through the fire and heal myself from that dark hole I somehow dug myself into, unintentionally. When I just didn't care anymore, I had to search for the light.

Burnout happened to me. It happened because of me. And it took work to get out of it.

And this is where The Enoughness Method comes in. It's from that deep, dark place of emptiness that the rebuilding of my life happened. It is a blend of self-care and nervous system recalibration techniques that moves the body from a sympathetic nervous system response into a parasympathetic nervous system response.

Whenever anxiety, feeling overwhelmed, or panic set in, I felt as though the tiger was closing in on my heels and I was running for my life. In reality, there was no tiger. My job wasn't related to life or death. I kept myself in a fight-or-flight response, which triggers the sympathetic nervous system, because I didn't know anything else. I didn't know better and when I burned out in 2013, research associating burnout to a reduced parasympathetic nervous system wasn't something I found.

I learned the hard way over the course of many years that my fight-or-flight response shut down the parasympathetic response. I figured out what actually worked for me and what felt good not only for my body, but what helped restore a sense of peace within.

Getting my body out of fight-or-flight took practice. It took time to get out of the habit of checking my email, responding to text messages, or tapping notifications on social media apps before I poured love into myself.

It was like I was addicted to burnout. I couldn't stop. It was easy for me to stay in the state of overdrive, go-go-go, anxiety, start work early, stay late, eat at my desk, skip social functions because I couldn't relate to anyone anymore.

The Enoughness Method gave me enough space to breathe deeper, think more clearly, and feel safer in my body. When that happened, I realized I was worthy of self-love and prioritizing myself and my mental health before I took on the day and daily tasks. And when the day got crazy, which they often did, I looked to my simple three-step process to help me calm down:

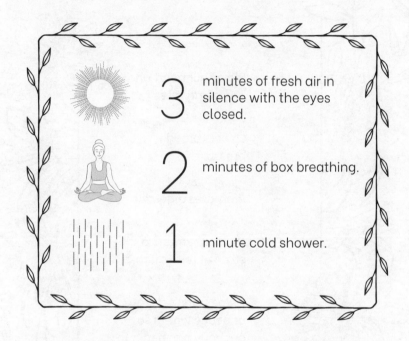

When COVID hit, I fell back into burnout, along with millions of other people. The second time through burnout was different. I knew I was in it. And I knew what I had to do to get out of it. I had to get myself outside. I knew I had to get myself into cold water. And I knew I had to get out of the house and away from everyone to meditate and take deep breaths.

The Enoughness Method taps into the parasympathetic nervous system because it hits all the high points necessary for burnout recovery.

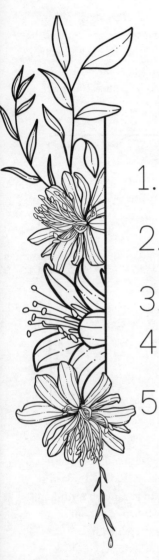

1. Slows our heart and breathing rates.

2. Lowers blood pressure.

3. Promotes digestion.

4. Our body enters a state of relaxation.

5. Helps us find a state of peace within so our body can begin to recover.

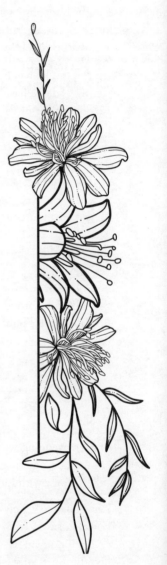

The Burnout Recovery Journey

It was early 2019. The latest download from the Universe was that I was to *Be the House*. I knew I had to create a publishing house. I had tools to burnout recovery I didn't have before. A lot of them. I knew how to calm myself down, get out of fight-or-flight, and move forward without spiraling downward.

I told myself that I could start another business. Within a matter of months I pieced together The Unapologetic Voice House, signed on my first seven book clients, and found a book distributor.

The word *unapologetic* was everywhere in my personal life. I encompassed the concept of being unapologetic in how I showed up in life. Fully myself. I had just turned 40. I was in a relationship I knew was for life. I had close to 100 rejection letters from agents telling me I wasn't enough for them. And I was tired of apologizing for not being someone or something else. I was wholeheartedly living unapologetically. I wanted to be in partnership with others who were unapologetic in their life experiences as well.

I officially started The Unapologetic Voice House in May 2019, and the first books were published in the Fall of 2019, just weeks after Gavin spontaneously asked me to be his wife on Friday, September 13, hours shy of the Harvest full moon making its yearly appearance.

Our engagement was different and even a bit clunky. Like us. And perfect. He proposed with a ninety-nine-dollar ring we picked out at a place called Crystal Magic. It was made with gold quartz, and I squealed like a little girl when I tried it on for the first time.

Our wedding was set for the Red Rocks of Sedona, Arizona. It was going to be a destination wedding for everyone, including us. I grew up in the Midwest with lots of family. Grandparents, loads of uncles, aunts, first cousins, second cousins, and whatever you call the children of the first and second cousins. We called everybody cousins.

Despite not seeing everyone every day, we kept in touch and knew everything about one another. My family was really good at the telephone game. As soon as someone got seriously injured, engaged, had their heart broken, won some sporting event, or lost one, within a few days, dozens and dozens and dozens of people knew what happened. That was the way we did life. It was normal. Expected.

Since our wedding was a destination wedding, my family made sure our guests always had things to do.

Guests who arrived on Friday got an invite to a couple's shower. Gavin and I were known for getting up and deciding that day that we needed a road trip. We'd pack up some clothes, the dog and her food, and stuff everything in the car and go. Where to and for how long was never discussed until the first red light we hit. So our couple's shower had an adventure theme. It was catered with food from Wisconsin, Arizona, Pennsylvania, and California. I grew up in Wisconsin and Gavin grew up partly in California and Pennsylvania. We expected eighty guests.

The next day, everyone was scheduled to drive up to Sedona. We rented out a picnic space from noon-to-sunset at Crescent Moon Picnic Site that was on Oak Creek, really close to where we got engaged, just under Cathedral Rock. We ordered food and planned on the same eighty people showing up to play all day with us. We considered it the groom's event and gave guests the night off to recover from being out in the sun all day.

The wedding was planned for the next day. We had yoga planned and hair and make-up for a ton of ladies. We expected 168 guests total. My brother turned 40 the day after the wedding, so we just kept the party going. Whoever was still there was invited to join us for fun events, like Jeep tours up the red rocks, hiking, and dinner. We planned for about forty guests to be there. Our honeymoon was scheduled to start the following weekend.

And then came spring break of 2020. We had Gavin's kids with us that year and since he and I used any excuse to get out of town, I suggested we go sledding up north. We piled the kids and dog into the car and popped up to Flagstaff for a quick road adventure. During the drive back to our house in Scottsdale on Friday, March 13, we talked about what everyone in the world was talking about.

COVID.

I refreshed every news app on my phone every few minutes to see the updates and I'd share it with Gavin.

Everything was unknown that week.

Are the kids going back to school?

Where are we going to find toilet paper?

How much food should we get?

And will our wedding extravaganza, planned for April 17–20, 2020, actually happen?

My heart ached every time he claimed our wedding would be canceled because of what was unfolding. Considering we had 168 people coming to the wedding itself but had three full days of events planned for guests, the thought of it all evaporating hurt deeply.

Gavin would have preferred to elope. But I made a promise to my mom when I was 16 that I would never do that. Or wear a red wedding dress. Or have a black ring for a wedding ring.

Being an optimistic person, as I read all the horrible news and listed out what was shutting down moment-by-moment, I leaned into everything I knew about visualization and kept seeing us at every party — including the wedding — with guests.

Before we got home, Gavin took a detour and drove to a supermarket to buy as much of everything in bulk as we could fit in the car.

On Sunday, the Governor ordered all schools to close for two weeks, giving parents an opportunity to prepare for at-home learning. I ordered computers for the kids and began turning our home into a makeshift pre-school so Gavin's youngest kid would be entertained and educated when with us.

The next morning, March 16, 2020, thirty-two days before our actual wedding, the Governor of Arizona released an executive order that stated special events, like weddings with more than ten guests, were banned from happening in the state of Arizona until further notice.

I saw the news break on social media as I sat at the kitchen table having coffee that Saturday morning. I read the mandate several times and couldn't believe it. I heard Gavin stir from the bedroom and told him what I knew. And then I called my mom. It felt like I was moving through water. I could see my feet moving but I couldn't feel them. I saw my hand in front of me tap the phone screen but couldn't register what was happening.

"The Governor shut down the wedding," I told my mom when she picked up the phone.

"I'm so sorry, honey. I'm so heartbroken for you," she said.

Heartbroken was a word I'd soon own, but right then in that moment I had stepped out of my body, so I didn't have to feel it.

What happened next was a bigger blur. While we spoke, an email from the wedding venue manager came through sharing the same news. And she included a variety of new dates for my wedding.

Not knowing how long the mandate would last, I selected a date in November and sent out an email to all our guests letting them know the bad news.

Like everyone else on the planet, I went through COVID the best I could, knowing full well I was back in burnout.

Gavin and I managed school online for his kids, teaching his youngest sight words with preschool educational books my sister gave us. We took turns being the teacher in the house, making sure everyone was doing what they were supposed to do during the school day. While he managed the kids and their education, I worked.

The Unapologetic Voice House grew fast in 2020. I signed on twenty new authors during 2020 and published books on a regular basis. The business was full and busy and when I wasn't managing something with the kids, I used my workload as a way to numb out from the wedding blues.

The reality of it was I let the wedding that never happened drag me down into a depression. It was all over me. I could feel it grab hold of my heart, my gut; my thoughts were cloudy.

I was one of a million-or-so expected brides managing the grief of a fairy-tale gone missing. My original wedding weekend came and went and nothing happened. Within a matter of months, I ate my way past several additional sizes and couldn't have squeezed into my wedding gown if I tried to.

When the overwhelming, ongoing stress of life was too much for me, I'd practice The Enoughness Method.

I'd lie outside in the grass under a tree and watch the leaves on the branches above me move in the breeze. I closed my eyes and practiced box breathing with the dog next to me. I started and ended my day with a cold shower.

In August 2020, another email came from the wedding venue that stated we had to postpone again because the mandate still wasn't lifted for events over ten individuals. Before I called my mom, I wrote a letter to God.

Dear God. This sucks. I'm tired of waiting. We live together. I'm helping raise his children. I don't want this grief anymore. Take it from me. What should I do?

Help me.

Carrie

As I waited for an answer, the heaviness of it all poured out of me. I couldn't catch my breath in between the wailing. I clenched my fists and pumped my fingernails into the palms of my hands, a trick I learned to break a thought or pattern. When I was able to inhale gulps of air, I took myself outside and sat down under the tree. I kicked my shoes off, laid back, and watched the clouds. With one hand on my belly and the other on my heart, I paid attention to my heartbeat. It was slowing down.

I closed my eyes and listened to the birds, the sensation of the grass on my legs, and the breeze drying my tears on my cheeks.

After a few minutes, I practiced my box breathing. And when I was ready, I went back inside, stripped down, and jumped in the shower before turning it on to the coldest I could.

I knew I couldn't control COVID or how it impacted most of life. What I could control though was staying single or getting married to my fiancé. I asked myself if I wanted to get married because of all the amazing events we planned, and replanned by that point, or did I want to be married to Gavin because he was my person?

He was my person. How it happened no longer mattered to me. It never mattered to him. All we needed was someone to marry us. People were having online weddings already. He and I could go somewhere out in the middle of nowhere and have someone marry us while everyone else watched online.

I ran the idea by Gavin. He loved being outdoors and didn't care how or when we got married. I shared my idea with my mom and she loved it. My new wedding plans took root and I went off to find a few cabins. It was so simple. And bittersweet still because of the plans that I lost.

Within a month, I found three cabins on the same street a few hours north from Phoenix. One house was for me, Gavin, and his kids. Another house was for my sister, her husband, and kids. The third house was for my parents, brother, and uncle. I found a baker, a florist, bought bride-tribe coffee cups and glass mugs that had our date on them. I bought a rose gold sequin dress online and sent out an invitation with an online meeting link to all the original guests.

The day before our weekend adventure took place we all took a test to ensure each of us were negative. We caravanned up north on Friday, two days before my wedding. My mom and I were in one car with my dress and Gavin's clothes, two coolers filled with snacks, wine, salmon, steaks, veggies, eggs, coffee creamer, and everything else my mother thought to pack. Gavin and the kids were in his car packed with suitcases that had play clothes, hiking gear, and toys for the kids. My sister, Holly, and her family came separately. My uncle, who ordained himself on the internet and agreed to manage the online meeting room as well as his duties as an officiant, drove himself. And my dad picked up my brother from the airport and they drove up together. My brother flew in from Pennsylvania and wore two masks on the plane. He refused to miss my wedding.

I stopped in Flagstaff to pick up cupcakes and our wedding cake before picking up my bouquet, wrist corsages for my mom and sister, and boutonniere for everyone else. Mom held the cake and cupcakes in her lap as we drove another thirty minutes down dirt roads until we found the cabins in the middle of the forest.

As we pulled into the pine needle crusted driveway, I rolled the windows down and took a deep breath. My body relaxed and I let out a squeal. All the disappointment and pain from plans unfulfilled didn't matter that weekend.

I was in the middle of nowhere getting married.

One by one the others rolled into the driveway of the main cabin where we would all be meeting. We had dinner together and went off in groups of two to go hiking, fishing, and exploring the following day. It was relaxing and enjoyable to finally be with family acknowledging my union with Gavin.

The morning of my wedding finally came. I woke up before everyone else and meditated with the moon still in the window. As the sun popped over the treetops, I took my coffee out on the back deck to get fresh air.

I sat there in silence, by myself, listening to the sounds of birds, pine cones falling, twigs breaking, and allowed the overwhelming sense of gratitude to wash over me time and time again.

Exhale.

Hold.

Inhale.

Hold.

After a while I went inside for my cold shower before chopping up vegetables. I made a big breakfast scramble and invited my family over to start the day together in celebration.

The day was beautiful. We took naps, played outside, and around two-thirty that afternoon, I went next door to the cabin where my mom and dad were staying to get ready with my sister.

Holly hung up my dress and took pictures of us getting ready with her phone. She did my hair and make-up and at four o'clock, we got in a line outside for our progression across the pine needles.

My uncle started the online meeting room and admitted everyone. We had music playing. Gavin and the kids were on the deck waiting. And right before we walked next door to meet Gavin on the deck, the dog got out.

There were thirteen people at my backwoods wedding ceremony held online on September 13, 2020, a year after we got engaged. And one dog.

There were moments throughout the ceremony where my uncle had to remind people to mute themselves. Gavin wiped tears from my cheeks, and I reached across to fasten a button he missed. Leia, our Goldendoodle, found a spot next to my brother. Gavin, the three kids, and I each poured our favorite candy into one big candy jar to signify the blending of us all as one family. My brother, dad, and stepson all read something. And my uncle surprised us by throwing fairy dust on us before he announced us husband and wife. It all happened in a matter of thirty minutes.

We never actually practiced how to signify the ceremony was complete. Normally, the couple walks off somewhere. After my uncle threw glitter on us and pronounced us hitched, Gavin took my hand and led me inside. He gently kissed me on my forehead.

"We're married," I laughed.

"I want to say hello to people who watched us online," he said.

I put my flowers back in the vase and grabbed a bottle of champagne from the refrigerator. Gavin took off his jacket and rolled up his sleeves. I poured champagne into a few glasses and handed one to Gavin before we walked back out on the deck to chat with everyone online.

We acknowledged everyone individually and thanked them for tuning in to our broadcast.

One by one, people signed off and we said goodbye.

We took a few photos out in the woods and on the dirt road leading to the cabin. When the sun started to set, my dad grilled steaks and salmon. He made a speech and so did my sister.

A few days later, we drove back home. Energetically, something shifted. There was a deeper sense of belonging within our relationship. I felt more connected to Gavin and was able to let go of the grief from the wedding extravaganza that never happened.

Gavin and I both stepped right back into our life together. The house was the same. The kids were still in school online, and we had a pretend preschool in the living room with sing-alongs, counting games, and sight words. The only difference was my last name.

I learned by that point that burnout doesn't stop overnight. It's a process and progress, and I needed to work my system to live my life in the way I really wanted.

At the end of 2020, I felt mostly settled. My unpublished book haunted me every time I turned my computer on. I had unfinished business with it and knew it was time to take inspired action.

The heartache of being compared to big-time authors dissipated. When I turned inward and questioned if publishing *Unapologetically Enough* myself was right, my eyes filled up with tears and angel bumps sprung up on my arms. A big, deep belly laugh came out of me. I yawned. I sighed. My body swayed back and forth. And I felt at complete peace within. It was divine timing.

Regardless of who I was compared to or what my book was compared to, I knew I couldn't keep it a secret any more.

Unapologetically Enough came out on the market in 2022 and the unknown of what strangers thought about it sent me on a wild roller coaster of emotions. The anxiousness that sat inside my body was familiar. I'd start my day with a cold shower, practice a breathing exercise, and meditate outside for a few minutes before coffee, Gavin, kids, or checking the status of orders, reviews, or new requests.

The feedback to *Unapologetically Enough* was unexpected. Readers called *Unapologetically Enough* a mental health book. Subscription boxes bought my book by the thousands to include in their monthly mental health and self-care boxes. Corporations and associations hired me to speak about burnout recovery and ways to improve morale in the workplace.

It was the speaking opportunities that gave me the chance to share my own unique burnout recovery method — The Enoughness Method — on stages in front of doctors, nurses, managers, program directors, executive directors, human resource, and information technology employees.

The more opportunities I called in to support people on their burnout recovery journey, the deeper down the research rabbit hole I fell. And it was thanks to the number of speaking engagements throughout 2023 that I learned just how burned out we all are and how many of us are also dealing with compassion fatigue, specifically, healthcare professionals, family caregivers, lawyers, non-profit leaders, and financial professionals.

Compassion fatigue isn't talked about as much in mainstream media, but it's important to look at. It comes on suddenly and is a result of having an empathic heart and being exposed to prolonged trauma, even if it's a client's trauma, which is why so many healthcare professionals are dealing with both compassion fatigue and burnout.

As I boarded a plane to head home after my last speaking engagement in 2023 to a big healthcare company, that big, flashing sign appeared again. This time, I didn't argue with it. I didn't flinch. I embraced it as my next stepping stone and created *The Enoughness Method: Reclaiming Your Power, Worth & Peace After Burnout.*

I finished it in perfect timing, too.

Gavin and I moved into a new home towards the end of 2023 and I loved our life together. Within a matter of two months, something was off for Gavin. His doctor ordered tests. It was just after Thanksgiving when Gavin's primary doctor left him a message and said, "I'm sorry to tell you, but the biopsy came back as malignant. We have to get on this."

Gavin forwarded that message to me, and I learned of his cancer sitting alone in a grocery store parking lot. I listened to the message over and over again. I thought of the faces of healthcare professionals in the audiences of speaking engagements over the last year. I knew they were swamped and stressed and burned out.

But to leave that message on his voicemail? I had things to say to that doctor.

As I punched in the last digit of that guy's number into my phone, I became acutely aware I was taking on a brand-new role.

I put on a cancer caregiver cape with matching medical advocate accessories.

I sat in on doctor appointments with Gavin, recorded conversations with his medical team so I could do my own research afterward, and joined cancer caregiver groups to support my own mental health.

It didn't take long for my nervous system to crack again and my body to remind me of what was at stake.

It wasn't just enough to take cold showers or sit outside or practice box breath. I practiced the exercises in this book, ones I had taught from the front of rooms to thousands of people and knew worked.

I navigated the caregiver role the same way I did the book, the business, the pandemic, and the nonprofit: with small, daily actions that reminded my mind, body, spirit, and nervous system, I am enough.

That's the who, what, how, and why of my burnout management and why I share *The Enoughness Method*. From here on out, let's work on yours.

Throughout the rest of this book, you'll find journal prompts, questions to help guide you through your own thought process behind why you are in burnout. You'll find checklists and additional tools to support your nervous system.

Take your time.

And before you start the rest, go outside for three minutes.

Exhale for four counts. Hold for four counts. Inhale for four counts. Exhale for four counts. Do it again three more times.

And jump in a cold shower for a minute.

You'll feel ready after that!

I love you.

Unapologetically.

PART II

The Narrative You Tell Yourself

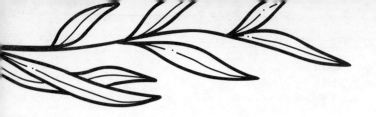

BEFORE I COULD reshape my life, I had to take a good look at myself and understand how I ended up burned out in the first place.

The truth was, I ended up in burnout because I was chasing money, accolades, and approval from others. I was in the trenches with thousands of other leaders killing myself for pennies. And if I won one, I was successful. The problem was, I had to prove myself every day in order to gain funds. It was toxic. And no matter how much money I gathered, I never felt full, satisfied, at home in my body and at peace because I couldn't ever take my armor off. There was always tomorrow, and the game started all over again. I was always fighting and never felt enough.

I kept myself in burnout because I took responsibility for everything in my business. I didn't pass along tasks to anyone else because I sucked at creating healthy boundaries for myself. I said yes to everything. I said yes to running workshops, speaking engagements, television segments, guest appearances here and there, fundraising, grant writing, mentoring, and the list went on and on.

Self-care was something I was really good at before I became an entrepreneur. I loved my list of self-care activities. And I thought I rocked self-care because I went places, spent money on myself, and exercised my heart out.

Before launching Severson Sisters, Saturdays were the days I would do an intense workout, go get my nails and toes done, go fill up on treats for myself, and sometimes go out, sometimes lie on the couch. Sundays were days I went to church and had dinner with family or friends, and that was it.

What I learned during my burnout recovery was that all my self-care activities supported my mental health. And all the things I did, the pedicures, hiking, and taking myself out for a treat or two, they were all acts that I hoped would lead me to a state of being.

That state of being was self-love. That took practice.

Self-love sometimes felt like a buzzword to me. It felt like a competition that I wasn't winning. It felt like I was doing self-love wrong because I never felt rejuvenated after something I thought was in the self-care bucket. Eventually, I assumed my peers were reading something I wasn't or watching something I wasn't.

There was shame involved in it.

I would see a post online from a woman living her best life in some beautiful home, in a bikini at a spa pool, or in some gorgeous setting with her friends or lover with something along the lines of "Filling up my cup" or "Work hard, play harder" or "Sunday Funday" in the caption. I'd think, *Once I can do that, I'll feel better about my life. My stress will be gone.*

I'd keep scrolling on some social media platform and see images of a woman doing some intense yoga move in the desert, looking totally at peace. I'd think, *I like the kind of yoga where you just lie there with your feet up the wall for like twenty minutes. Maybe I should try doing that kind of yoga, and I'll find peace within.*

After I launched the nonprofit, I didn't have time for self-care. I felt empty for years and knew something was missing. I just didn't love myself enough to stop working, protect my time and mental health, and make a shift. Until that is, the morning of my 35th birthday when I got a message from the Universe that I was a burnout.

After the morning I made a deal with myself to heal my burnout, everything in my life revolved around self-care.

I considered a long nap an act of self-care.

I carved out time in my calendar to daydream.

I'd go on walks around a lake just to sit on my favorite bench and pretend tree roots grew out of my feet so I could feel more connected to Earth.

Watching clouds roll by, giving gratitude while standing in lines at grocery stores, or coffee shops, and even stopping to look at flowers all became part of my day. And I blocked out time in my calendar to do it.

I recreated my life around my self-care practices because I wanted to get out of burnout.

I realized that I welcomed a deeper level of happiness—both personal and professional. I was able to see that in order to move through my professional life happily, I first had to move through my overall life happily. And I've worked on myself enough to know that to bring about personal happiness, I first had to understand the feeling of happiness at a deeper level.

Throughout 2014, I focused on *activities* I knew would make me *feel* happy on a personal level. I trusted that when I moved from a place of

personal happiness, everything I did professionally would mirror my personal life.

My 2014 personal-happiness action-item list looked like this:

- Dance parties in the living room.
- Read more funny books.
- Go on more road trips.
- Cuddle animals.
- Play in the ocean.
- Wear fairy wings.
- Go to events with friends.
- Watch the clouds while lying in the grass.
- Meditate to pretty music.

Redefining success was deeply connected to the feeling of happiness and doing things that made me happy.

When I went back to work after my burnout, I set boundaries for myself, probably for the first time. Boundaries helped me be able to create more time in my day for my mental health. I started with work boundaries and that helped me shape my personal time.

I wouldn't take calls until nine o'clock. As the boss, I could do that. I woke up without an alarm, and again as the boss I could do that. I'd meditate after my coffee and go for a walk before looking at my phone.

I blocked off thirty minutes in my calendar every day for lunch. And I would go outside for lunch, when weather permitted.

I deleted social media and my email from my phone and stopped working at 5:30 every night.

And the biggest boundary was on the weekend. I didn't check my email until Monday morning again.

Getting out of burnout took time. And not just a long weekend. It took years. Burnout is a condition that we have to treat as seriously as we do diabetes or ADHD. It's something that won't go away on its own.

In this next section, you will want to take your time and get totally honest with yourself. Here's the hard truth and the tough love. You are in burnout because of neglecting your boundaries, your self-care routine, and your priorities. You're going to create boundaries around your time, your physical health, your mental health, your office, and your home life.

Remember, I love you.

Unapologetically.

And I was in your shoes a wee little bit ago.

Use this section to really look at your life, both at work and at home, and your habits, priorities, and attitude.

Before you start, though, go sit outside for three minutes. Do two min-utes of box breathing and stick your face in cold water for a minute.

Feel better?

Ok!

Ready...

3, 2, 1...

Here we go.

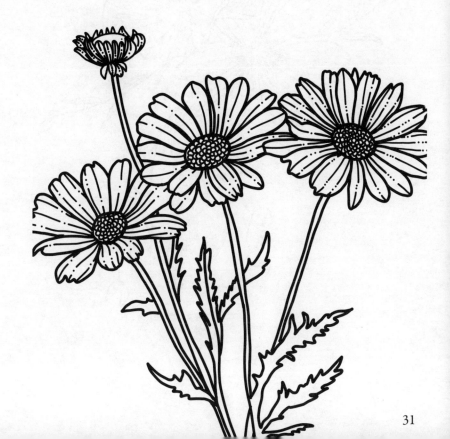

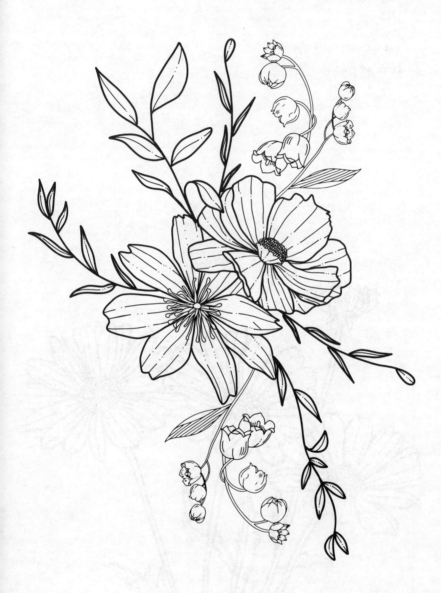

Personal Assessments, Daily Quizzes & Checklists

Below you'll find a few checklists and assessments.

First things first, let's check to see if you are hanging out with compassion fatigue or burnout or both! It can happen. You can be burned out AND suffering from being overly compassionate and having nothing left to give!

Check the boxes for symptoms you relate to in both compassion fatigue and burnout. This can be a daily, weekly, or monthly personal assessment.

Next, take a snapshot of the self-compassion checklist and check in with it daily. If these daily self-compassion tasks don't feel aligned with you, create your own in the space provided.

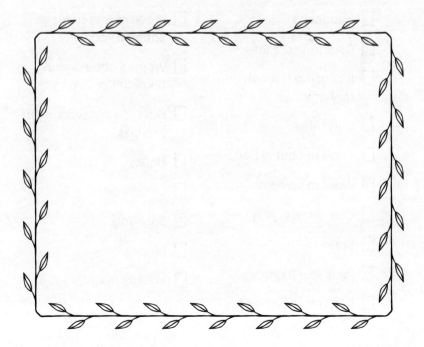

Where Am I Today?

- ☐ Compassion Fatigue
- ☐ Burnout
- ☐ Unable to balance empathy & objectivity
- ☐ Anxiety
- ☐ Difficulty focusing
- ☐ Bitter

- ☐ Negative outburst
- ☐ Weight gain
- ☐ Coasting till the end of day
- ☐ Apathy
- ☐ Hopelessness
- ☐ Resentful

How Do I Feel Today?

- ☐ Anxiety in my belly
- ☐ Headache
- ☐ Couldn't care less
- ☐ Just going through the motions
- ☐ Can't sleep
- ☐ Can't get out of bed
- ☐ Want to scream
- ☐ Can't stop crying
- ☐ Hopeful
- ☐ Ready for a change
- ☐ Better than yesterday

- ☐ Worse than ever before
- ☐ Proud of myself for eating a veggie
- ☐ Worried about setting boundaries
- ☐ Guilty for not wanting to exercise
- ☐ Happy
- ☐ Clearheaded
- ☐ Brain fog
- ☐ Relaxed
- ☐ In flight/flight/freeze

Self-Compassion Checklist

- ☐ Good quality sleep
- ☐ Did daily self-assessments
- ☐ Brown paper bag lunch
- ☐ Connected with a loved one
- ☐ Fifteen minutes of physical movement
- ☐ Named one win from the day
- ☐ Practiced The Enoughness Method at least once today
- ☐ Let myself have ten minutes of restorative relaxation
- ☐ Recognized my empathy boundary
- ☐ Left desk during breaks

My Own Self-Compassion Checklist

- ☐ _____
- ☐ _____
- ☐ _____
- ☐ _____
- ☐ _____

How did you end up in burnout?

In the space below, write your story of how you ended up in burnout.

_____

_____

_____

_____

_____

What do you feel are your responsibilities at work currently?

_____

_____

_____

_____

Why do you feel you're responsible for it?

_____

_____

_____

_____

Is there anyone else at work who can take on some of your responsibilities? If no, write down all the reasons why not. If YES, write down all the reasons why!!

_____

_____

_____

_____

_____

Name as many people as you can who can help you with any responsibilities that are not really yours.

_____

_____

_____

_____

What did you want to accomplish in your career when you first started?

_____

_____

_____

_____

What would you like to still accomplish in your career?

_____

_____

_____

_____

_____

_____

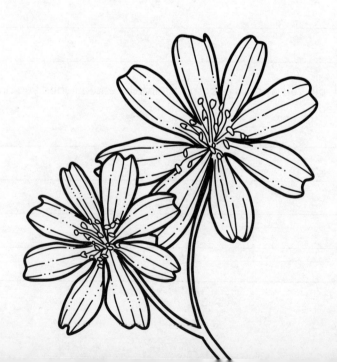

Letter of Personal Guidelines
While at Work

Dear _____,

I am a kind and caring individual. I have a huge heart and love to be of service. With that being said, I also recognize I am in need of some TLC, self-compassion, and balance.

Moving forward, I will conduct myself to my patients and colleagues with the utmost respect. I will be mindful of my words, attitude, time, and energy. I am capable of being a gracious leader in my field and know I make an impact and contribution with my skills. I will...

_____

_____

_____

_____

_____

_____

_____

_____

_____

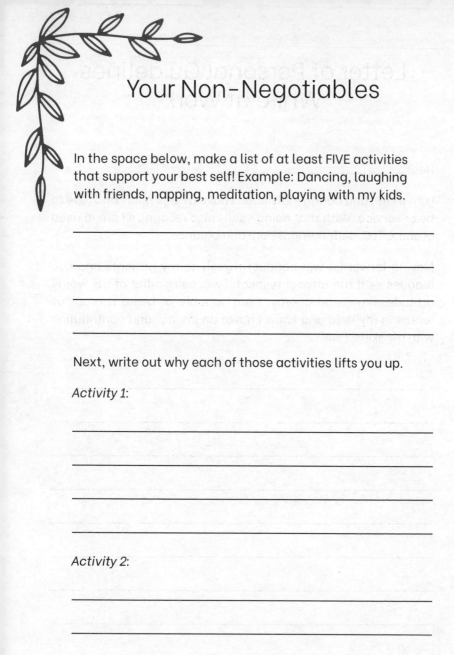

Your Non-Negotiables

In the space below, make a list of at least FIVE activities that support your best self! Example: Dancing, laughing with friends, napping, meditation, playing with my kids.

_____

_____

_____

Next, write out why each of those activities lifts you up.

Activity 1:

_____

_____

_____

_____

Activity 2:

_____

_____

_____

_____

Activity 3:

_____

_____

_____

Activity 4:

_____

_____

_____

_____

Activity 5:

_____

_____

_____

_____

Congratulations! You just made your list of Non-Negotiables!

Those five activities are what you now create boundaries around.

Protect those suckers as though your life depended upon it! Because it does!

Your Belief System

Before you look at *how* you can move, delete, or add things in your life to incorporate these non-negotiables you just admitted to yourself, I'd like you to first look at a few belief systems of yours.

Don't think about these questions too long. Answer them off the hip. Whatever comes first is your true answer.

Do you believe you deserve to come out of burnout?

_____

Do you feel ready to make a change in your life?

_____

Do you believe self-care is important?

_____

Do you accept the responsibility of prioritizing your self-care?

_____

Are you willing to practice The Enoughness Method at least once a day?

_____

If you answered no to any of these questions, head on over to my website and contact me. I'm serious. I want to talk to you, especially about that last one.

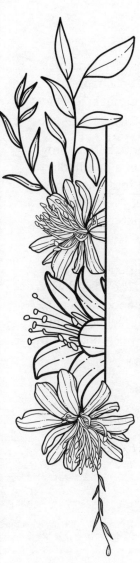

As a fellow burnout, I understand that it can feel scary to make a change. Also as a fellow burnout, I guarantee you that if you don't change, you're facing much more serious health concerns down your road.

So call me. Or email me. Whatever's easier for you.

Love you!

Unapologetically.

Moving on...

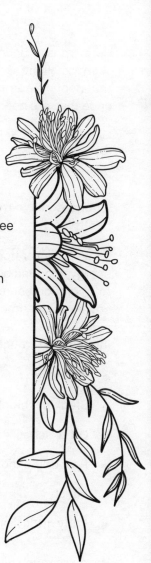

Creating Boundaries in Life

Here we are! Boundaries. Isn't this just the worst? Boundaries seem so cliche. And still, they are a big, grown-up whooptydoo that nobody learned in school but everyone figures out in real life once they are needed.

I was not good at boundaries until burnout. Prior to burnout, my boundaries involved blocking people on my phone and finding new coffee shops to hang out in. And truth be told, those two things are still in my boundary wheelhouse. But I've added additional tools to my belt over the years that support my mental health.

If you've never had to stand up for your mental health, time, or energy, creating boundaries can seem daunting. The easiest way to approach boundaries is to start with your calendar. Since recovery takes time, you'll have to examine your schedule and what needs to be adjusted. Our time is pretty much broken up into blocks throughout the day.

- Coffee time
- Breakfast block
- Off to school/work
- Rest of the morning
- Lunch
- Early afternoon
- Snacktime
- Late afternoon
- After work/school
- Dinner
- Bedtime

We do so much during the day. Within all that time, we're checking email, text messages, our social media accounts, the news, returning calls, making calls, keeping babies upright and accident free, driving to work, to school, to baseball, dance class, or music lessons, we're grocery shopping, volunteering, mowing lawns, picking up dog poop, house chores, feeding kids, spouses, kissing people, doing more than kissing people, napping, and working.

Did I miss anything?

Research on burnout changes all the time. The number of people who reported feeling burned out fluctuated based on the study. Some studies done in 2022 report close to 80% of Americans were burned out. Other studies looked at burnout industry to industry.

Regardless, the big lesson about recovery is that it will not happen in a single day. You will have to take small steps and accept small victories every day. Working your self-care, non-negotiables, and The Enoughness Method into your daily routine is necessary and so, to stay committed to it, calendar blocking is also necessary.

I have a few more questions for you to put some thought into. It's important that you take your time to answer these because these two questions will help your recovery journey.

Are you willing to get up six minutes earlier every day to practice The Enoughness Method before you leave for work, get the kids up, let the dog out, or look at your phone?

☐ YES	☐ NO

Are you willing to avoid looking at your email or social media before you get ready for the day (including practicing The Enoughness Method)?

☐ YES	☐ NO

Are you willing to avoid looking at your work email after work?

☐ YES	☐ NO

Are you willing to put your phone down and leave it alone after a certain time every night?

☐ YES	☐ NO

If you didn't answer YES to all those questions, head over to my website and shoot me an email. I want to talk about this.

If you answered YES to all of those questions, keep going!

I love you!

Unapologetically!

Moving on...

Let's look a bit more at your calendar. I have three bold recommendations for you to make when it comes to burnout recovery and your calendar.

1. Block off your lunch break, whether it's ten minutes or an hour, in your calendar. Every day, Monday through Friday, whenever you take a break for lunch, block it off on your calendar so nobody can book a call or request a meeting with you during a specific time every day. I understand some professions can't block off specific time every day because their breaks happen around patients. For those professionals, I recommend using your break time wisely by practicing The Enoughness Method. However, if you can schedule your lunch break, block it off.

2. Block off two fifteen-minute blocks through each day for human stuff. Get up. Stretch your legs. Do The Enoughness Method. Call your mom. Do a little dance party.

   Your time is valuable and taking a fifteen-minute break twice a day for human behavior is really healthy. I recommend fifteen-minutes mid-morning and fifteen-minutes mid-afternoon.

3. Creating boundaries around your time is to avoid scheduling calls or meetings before or past a certain time. If you aren't in the office until 8:15 every day, don't schedule a call at 8:15. If you are able to leave at 5 p.m. every night, don't schedule a meeting at 4:45 p.m. Take ownership of your calendar and make others do the same.

Now, let's look at your calendar. What's one task you eliminate or pass along to someone else so you have more space in your day?

☐ Blocked off my calendar for lunch every day.

☐ Blocked off a fifteen-minute morning human break.

☐ Blocked off a fifteen-minute afternoon human break.

☐ Committed to owning my calendar and booking meetings on my schedule.

Now that you're owning your precious time, you're going to look at *how* you can start to adjust where you spend your time.

In the space below, rewrite your five new non-negotiables you decided upon in the previous section.

1. _____

2. _____

3. _____

4. _____

Example: I can ask someone else to get birthday treats for the office. I can say no to weekly update meetings when my projects don't have updates. I can ask my son to walk the dog around the block. I can ask my spouse to unload and load the dishes.

_____

_____

_____

_____

Next, name one non-negotiable that can enter that free space!

Example: With my new free thirty-minutes before work, I can go for a walk before I leave in the morning. During the day, I can have a call with my mom on my lunch break. I can go to a knitting group after work. I can get up twenty minutes earlier to meditate. I can find an online dance class I can do in my living room.

_____

_____

_____

_____

Protect Your Boundaries

This was probably the hardest exercise for my own growth. As we accept the fact that we have to make changes in our lives for our lives to actually change, our circle of influence needs to be looked at.

Being able to recognize whom I had let go from my day-to-day life for the sake of my mental health, well-being, and overall growth was not easy. I had created pockets of friends, acquaintances, and colleagues I could turn to. But they weren't the best for the highest good.

I decided to put energy into the people in my life I knew, without a doubt, wanted the best for me. I focused on them. I gave gratitude for them in my daily journal entries. I sent them sweet-little-nothing messages or a funny story from my day. I stopped nurturing relationships that were one-sided or not in alignment with my healing. And soon, my life started to shift. People who weren't helping me find my highest good started to create distance from me and me from them. It happened naturally.

I said no to invitations to events happening during my self-care hours. And I started inviting people I wanted to spend more time with out for walks, hikes, or even meet-ups at the dog park.

I didn't have to have long drawn-out conversations with people. I started my boundaries with a few folks who drained my energy by simply imagining the line of connection between my heart, stomach, and mind being cut from their heart, stomach, and mind.

From there, I shared my plans to put energy into my self-care and that meant to no longer be available for texting or calls between certain hours of the day and week. Let's start with the tricky part. People who are not in alignment with our highest good are ones you'll want to create a boundary around and start to distance yourself from. Knowing WHO to create a boundary from is key.

Boundaries can be energetic, physical, or emotional, and sometimes a combination of them all. They protect our mental and
physical health, and it is a form of self-care to create them and
stick to them.

In this section, you'll fill in the blanks with names of people in your
daily life.

After I have a conversation with

_____, I feel depleted.

When I see _____ coming down the
hallway, I get a knot in my stomach.

When _____ calls me, I don't want
to pick up because I know it will be a draining
conversation.

_____ makes me want to cry.

I always get a headache when _____
and I chat.

I don't feel like I can support

_____'s drama anymore.

The individuals named in the previous exercise are a good starting point for where to create boundaries. If you are feeling physically, mentally, or emotionally impacted in a negative way by individuals in your daily life, it's time to make a change.

Boundaries can start with a simple energetic shift in your own behavior. Imagine a cord between yourself and a person listed in the previous section. Now imagine a sword slicing the cord in two.

Next, in the section below, prepare a statement outlining your boundary so you have it ready to go when you need it.

Examples are:

I love our chats, but I need to focus on my productivity so I can complete everything and leave on time.

I will check in on this tomorrow.

I'm putting my phone on airplane mode now for the rest of the day.

I need to put my energy elsewhere right now.

These are all great one-liners. And they can be used in all sorts of situations. Burnout is typically a professional issue. My experience is that it crept over into my personal life. I couldn't take on one more thing. I didn't want to be re-sponsible for keeping track of anything else, so I used these one-liners with family members. However, they knew I was struggling and were much easier to talk to about my boundaries than anyone in my professional life.

Boundaries are personal. They are strong statements that are meant to be clear and final.

Use "I" statements and remember how powerful the words "I AM" are when used together, so be sure not to claim something negative, heavy, or hard as your own here. AVOID statements like:

I am too overwhelmed right now to take on anything else.

I am unable to do that.

I am about to snap.

What I've learned about burnout is that it impacts men and women of all ages. It does not discriminate. An individual making $40,000 a year can be burned out and the person making $400,000 a year can also be burned out. Boundaries are used to help each person move one step further from that burnout swamp. Use them well.

What can you say to create a clear boundary between you and any one person listed in the previous section?

_____

_____

_____

_____

_____

Now, let's move on to the good stuff!

Write down three individuals in your daily life who support your highest good.

1. _____

2. _____

3. _____

And now write down why you feel supported by each.

Example: I feel supported by my boss. She goes out of her way to point out what I'm doing right in my job, and that lifts my spirits. Feeling recognized for what I do makes me feel proud.

1. _____

   _____

   _____

2. _____

   _____

   _____

3. _____

   _____

   _____

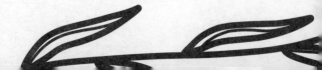

Next, it's important to acknowledge your own actions. How do you respond in each of the scenarios you listed?

Example: When I feel supported by my boss, I come home feeling happier and have energy to go for a walk with the dog.

1. _____

   _____

   _____

   _____

2. _____

   _____

   _____

   _____

3. _____

   _____

   _____

   _____

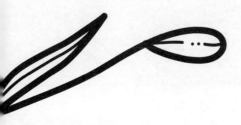

What can you do to show gratitude for the people you listed in the previous section?

Examples: Picture each person in a bright bubble and say THANK YOU out loud. Invite someone to coffee or lunch. Send a checking-in text. Make this super simple so you actually follow through!

_____

_____

_____

_____

_____

_____

_____

_____

_____

_____

_____

Elimination Tank

In order to see my burnout as a blessing, I first leaned into any personal traits or habits of mine that lead to burnout in the first place.

Get honest with yourself here. Nobody's looking. Circle the emotions below that you recognize within yourself.

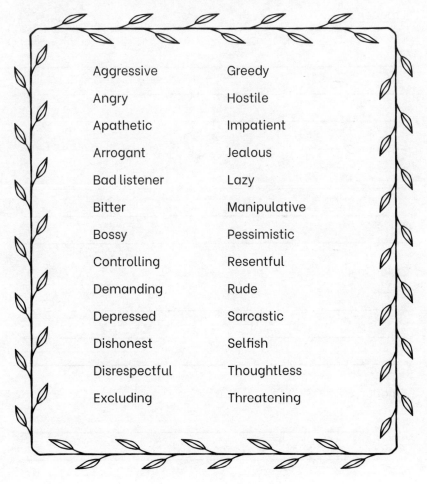

Aggressive	Greedy
Angry	Hostile
Apathetic	Impatient
Arrogant	Jealous
Bad listener	Lazy
Bitter	Manipulative
Bossy	Pessimistic
Controlling	Resentful
Demanding	Rude
Depressed	Sarcastic
Dishonest	Selfish
Disrespectful	Thoughtless
Excluding	Threatening

Select one emotion at a time. In the space below, write what comes to you when you ask yourself this question: Why am I showing up this way?

Emotion 1:

_____

_____

_____

Emotion 2:

_____

_____

_____

Emotion 3:

_____

_____

_____

Emotion 4:

_____

_____

_____

Emotion 5:

_____

_____

_____

Do you think it's important to show up differently? Why or why not.

_____

_____

_____

_____

Are there emotions you no longer wish to claim as your own? Why?

_____

_____

_____

_____

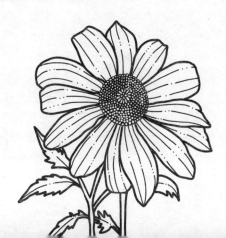

Use this as a time to identify anything you see in yourself that you wish to change.

_____

_____

_____

_____

_____

_____

_____

_____

_____

_____

_____

_____

_____

_____

_____

_____

_____

What is the EXACT opposite of each emotion?

Example: The opposite of jealousy could be appreciation.

Emotion 1: _____

The opposite is: _____

Emotion 2: _____

The opposite is: _____

Emotion 3: _____

The opposite is: _____

Emotion 4: _____

The opposite is: _____

Emotion 5: _____

The opposite is: _____

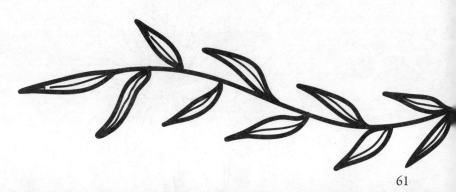

What must change in your life in order for you to show up as the opposite?

_____

_____

_____

_____

_____

Are you willing to have honest conversations with your friends and family about the changes you've committed to make?

☐ YES   ☐ NO

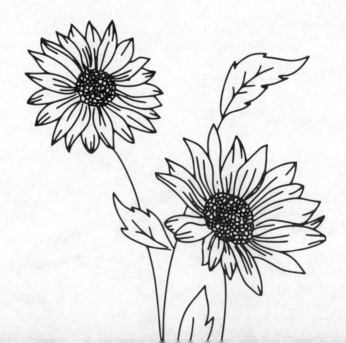

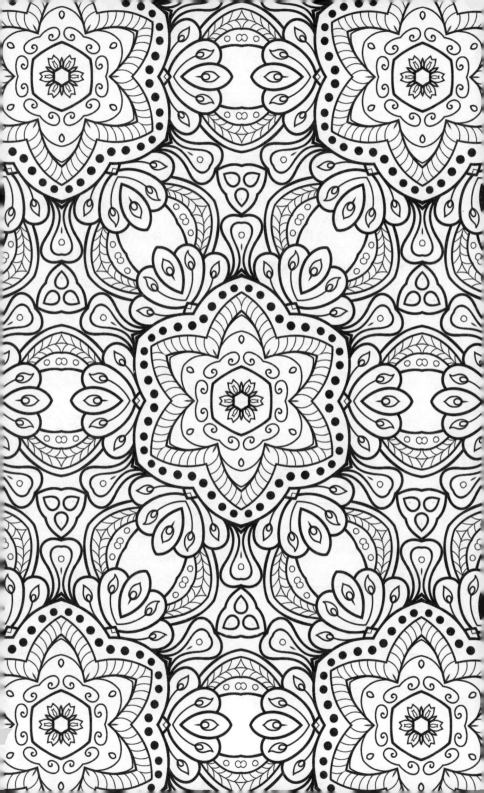

I AM . . .

These two words are powerful. I filled my journals with affirmations, mantras, and prayers that all started with the words I AM. They are important. What I found is, at first, they were just words. I didn't recognize the power they held because I couldn't feel it. That is, until I started to connect feelings and actions to them. After a while of doing these exercises, I recognized a shift within.

In the space below, write out five I AM statements that you believe about yourself today. Make them positive and believable.

Examples: I AM loving and feel safe. I AM capable and believe in myself. I AM open for a change and ready to commit to my burn-out recovery.

1. _____

_____

_____

_____

2. _____

_____

_____

_____

3. _____

_____

_____

_____

_____

4. _____

_____

_____

_____

_____

5. _____

_____

_____

_____

_____

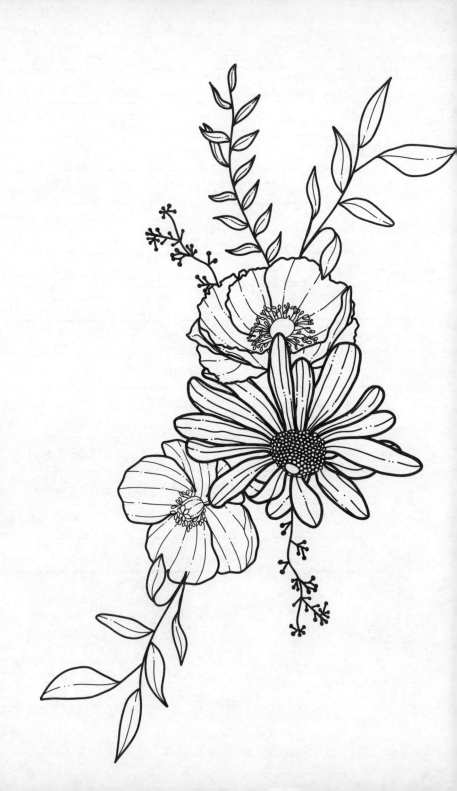

PART III

The Nervous System

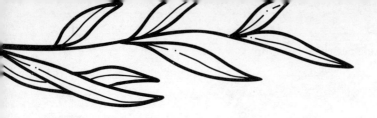

IF YOU'RE IN a state of burnout, the sympathetic nervous system has activated your fight-or-flight response. The sympathetic nervous system isn't all bad. It is there to keep everyone alive. Besides that, I'm personally not a big fan of my sympathetic nervous system. I imagine you aren't either.

The sympathetic nervous system increases heart rate, impacts your ability to poop (as in you don't go), makes you sweat more, raises your blood pressure, and a bunch of other gross things.

With every bad is good. With all the dark is light. It's that way with our nervous system, too.

The nervous system has this big nerve associated with it called the vagus nerve. It starts in the brain, runs down behind the ears, down the throat, into the belly, and touches all sorts of organs including the heart, reproductive organs, liver, lungs, and bladder.

Recovery from burnout has a lot to do with this vagus nerve. When it's activated, it sends signals out that YES... all is well in the world.

I am good.

I am at peace.

I am relaxed.

And when the vagus nerve is activated, all sorts of good things happen. Blood pressure decreases. Quality sleep increases. A state of relaxation takes place. And the most important thing that happens is related to the parasympathetic nervous system.

That's the good one. I want to be in that state as often as possible. When I'm in a parasympathetic state, my life flows better.

The Enoughness Method activates the vagus nerve three different ways.

3 minutes outside in fresh air.

2 minutes of box breathing.

1 minute cold shower.

But getting ourselves into a parasympathetic state can happen in a number of other ways. Check out other ways to recalibrate your nervous system in this section. And grab the download of all of these on the website.

Download The Enoughness Method Accessory on my website!

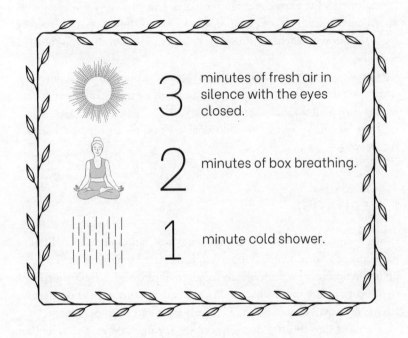

3 minutes of fresh air in silence with the eyes closed.

2 minutes of box breathing.

1 minute cold shower.

10 Additional Ways to Reset
the Nervous System

In addition to The Enoughness Method of 3, 2, 1, where you utilize stillness and silence in fresh air, box breathing, and a cold shower, there are plenty more techniques to help your nervous system shift out of an overstimulated response.

I'm not a doctor or a scientist. I'm a recovering burnout. Sometimes just a plain 'ol burnout. The tips offered in this book are from experience at carving my own path through burnout.

Here are my favorite 10 additional techniques to support burnout recovery:

1. MEDITATION

I am a big meditator. I have been practicing meditation since 2006. I found it because of a horse named Bubba. Bubba threw me into a tree and I wound up in physical therapy with a really tough therapist. She recommended I go to hot yoga before my sessions so she could dig into my muscles deeper and stretch my psoas. I hated Bubba after learning about the psoas muscle.

I walked into the 104-degree room for my first hot yoga class and sat down next to a woman who looked about my age. She smiled at me and asked if I was there for a spiritual awakening. It was the first time I heard the term. I didn't want to seem out of place, so I smiled back and nodded.

After class, I drove over to a bookstore and asked the clerk behind the information desk where I would go to find books about spiritual awakenings. She leaned in and whispered, "In the New Age section."

I ended up hunkered down in the corner of the New Age section row, which was only a single row back then, and read everything I could about meditation before my eyes got tired. I was hooked. I bought CDs with different meditation styles and listened to my first guided meditation that night on my living room floor.

Meditation is a great tool to use when I am in fight-flight because it tells my mind, body, gut, and spirit that I am safe. And my nervous system moves over to the parasympathetic one. I'm not alone in that miracle. It will happen for you, too.

If you're new to meditation, start by playing music that will help you slow your breath, release your muscles, and feel safe. I love using high vibrational music I find online known as the Solfeggio frequencies. There are nine different scales, and they are all beneficial and have their individual purposes. Some days I listen to 432Hz; other days I listen to 999Hz. I know it's the right tone and tune after a few minutes because my body will start to sway.

Look up Solfeggio frequencies and listen to a few different songs until you find one that works with your nervous system. Close your eyes, take deep breaths, and let yourself move out of fight-flight and into a state of relaxation.

What high vibrational frequency works best for your body right now?

_____

How did it feel listening to it?

_____

When can you make time in your day to meditate?

_____

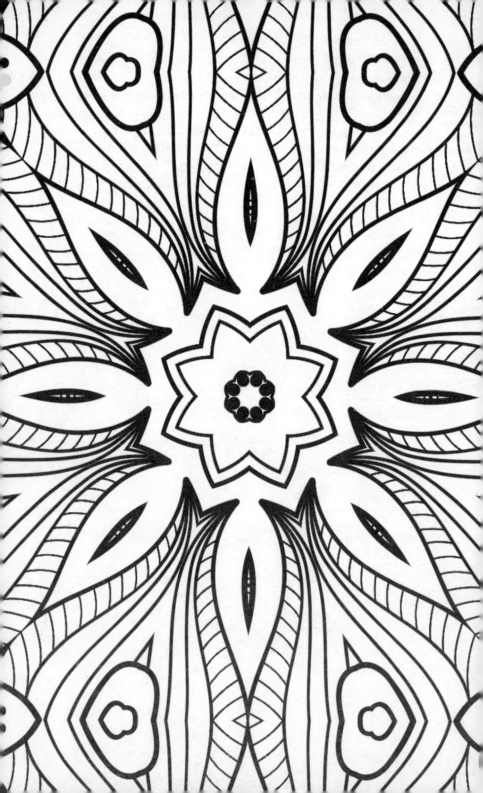

2. HAVENING

I found this technique later in my journey. A self-care technique I used early on in my journey was to stand in the mirror and talk lovingly to myself. And when I cried, I'd hug myself. Eventually, I would start to sway, and I wondered why. Through research, I found this self-soothing technique called Havening Touch™. There are practitioners all around the world teaching this method.

Havening is simply a soft, soothing touch.

To haven, cross your arms over your chest and lightly run your hands down your arms to your elbows and then back up to the tops of your shoulders. As you lightly run your hands down your arms, say powerful I AM statements out loud. Examples are:

I am safe.

I am peaceful.

I am supported.

Do this a few dozen times until the feeling of being overwhelmed subsides and you start to relax. While it's not necessary to do this standing in front of a mirror, I found it helped me really connect to it, and that acknowledgment moved me into parasympathetic mode quicker.

Go try it and come back!

How does it feel to practice havening?

_____

What is your power statement for this technique?

_____

3. 4-7-8 BREATH

This is a breathing technique I teach in burnout recovery workshops. I appreciate this breathing pattern because I have to stay focused on it. It's harder to get lost in thought when each round has three different counts.

For this one, inhale for four counts. Hold for seven counts. Exhale for eight counts and when you exhale, pretend you're blowing up a balloon. Make the whooshing sound with your breath.

Repeat this breathing pattern four times through. As you get used to this one, you'll want to increase how many times you do it. At first, you might be lightheaded, so don't do this one while driving!

This is a great technique to do when you start to feel anxiety creep in or your fight-flight response is crowding you. Four rounds of this technique takes just over a minute. Take ninety seconds to yourself somewhere private and give yourself four rounds of 4-7-8.

How does it feel after you perform four rounds of 4-7-8?

_____

Can you feel a difference in your body and, if so, where?

_____

When can you make time in your day to perform this exercise?

_____

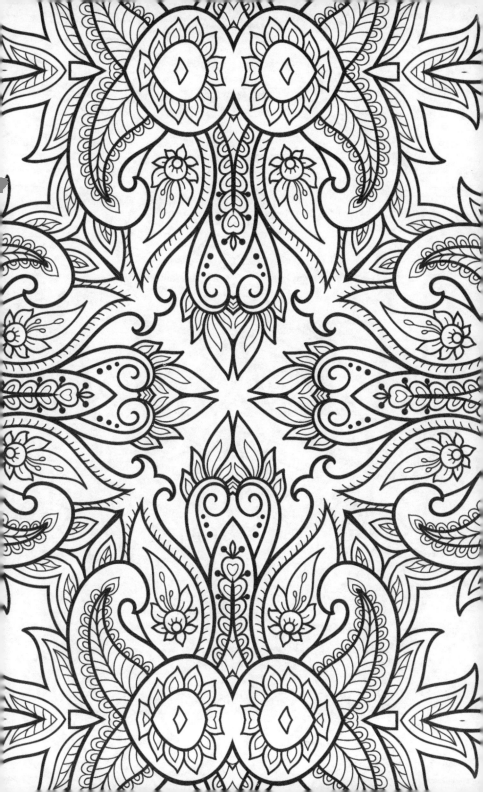

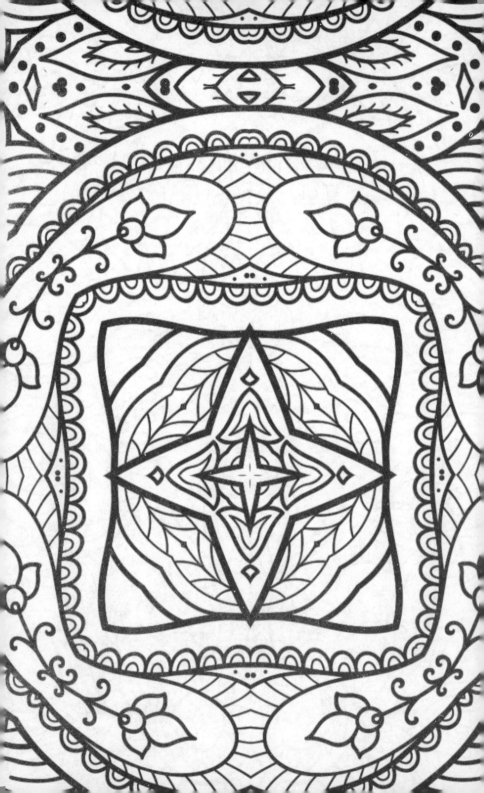

4. TAPPING

I've done this for a long time. This is also called emotional frequency technique (EFT). I love being guided through a tapping session by a coach. I always have a big ugly cry when I'm done doing this. So ye be warned.

There are points on the body called acupoints. By lightly tapping on certain points on your hands, face, and body while thinking about a certain issue, you're disrupting your thoughts and telling your body you are safe and at home in your body. The idea is that by tapping, you reduce the anxiety around that thought. There are several points on your body you can tap:

- The side of the hand
- Above the eyebrow
- On the side of the eye
- Underneath the eye
- Under the nose
- Under the lips
- Collarbone
- Under the armpit
- On top of the head

As you tap on various points of your body, admit to yourself that you have a concern. And then also admit to yourself that you are safe, and remind yourself that you love you!

The script for this technique goes like this: Even though I have (write in a concern you have)

_____ ,

I love and accept myself.

Every practitioner is different with this technique in terms of how many rounds to perform. I find it easiest to do it four times through and always start with the side of the hand and end with the top of the head.

What's great about this self-soothing technique is that it doesn't have to be done standing up, it doesn't make a lot of noise, and can be done with small movements so people sitting around you may not even notice. It might just look like you have an itch on your face!

Where did you notice a shift in your energy with this tool?

_____

5. HUMMING

I do this in the car. It works. Give it a shot.

Humming activates the vagus nerve in the body. So, think of a nursery rhyme. Any of them will do. Maybe you like Twinkly stars, or Mary and her sheep, or you're into Bonnie and the sea. Personally, my go-to is Happy Birthday! I'll sing it with my name or that of family members or friends, and just keep repeating it!

Got your tune? Now, hum it for several minutes over and over again. Go on, try it! Hum right now. Touch your fingertips to the side of your neck, close to your jaw line. Can you feel it vibrate? You activated your vagus nerve! Congrats! Your little diddy just told your heart, gut, brain, and a bunch of other pieces of you that you are in a safe state and all is well.

What tune did you hum?

_____

How do you feel after you hummed for a few minutes?

_____

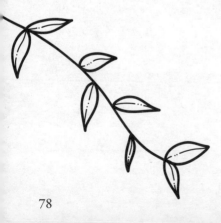

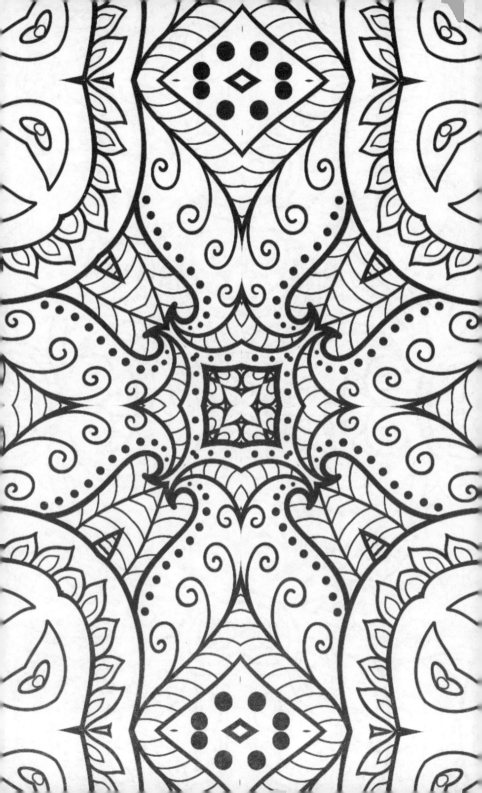

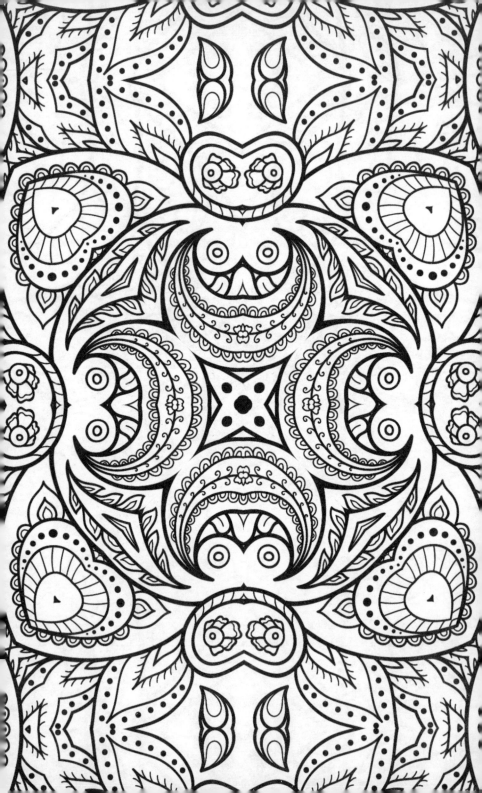

6. SINGING

Again with the vagus nerve, baby! This one works everywhere!
Sing while you're at the park, walking the dog, cooking dinner,
doing chores, in the car, even in the shower! Go on and belt it out!
Nobody's judging you.

When I'm in the car and have the radio on, I'll sing songs I know.
While I was in burnout, I preferred to have silence in the car. The
added noise increased my anxiety. Singing is something I'll do as
I'm sitting at my computer waiting for my next meeting to start.

My go-to for this is Happy Birthday, too! Typically I'll sing a few
rounds with my name in the verse and then I'll hum it.

What song did you sing?

_____

How do you feel after singing a few verses?

_____

7. SIGHING

I worked with a naturopath throughout my original stint with burnout, and she noticed I sighed a lot. Like a lot a lot. She asked me if I felt a sense of relief when I sighed. I never did, actually. I felt like I couldn't exhale hard enough which is why I sighed so much. She suggested I try sighing with a big AHHHH sound.

Take a deep breath and release it slowly with a big sigh. Pretend you're in a yoga class and be that person in class who isn't afraid to make the erotic noises. It's good for you. Nobody's watching! Let it go! Do it a few times in a row. After a while, you won't notice you're sighing with sound!

Sighing calms your mind, lowers your blood pressure, and will help with releasing anxiety and sadness from your body.

How does your body feel after a few sound sighs?

_____

Are you embarrassed to sound sigh?

_____

Who do you think is judging you and why?

_____

_____

_____

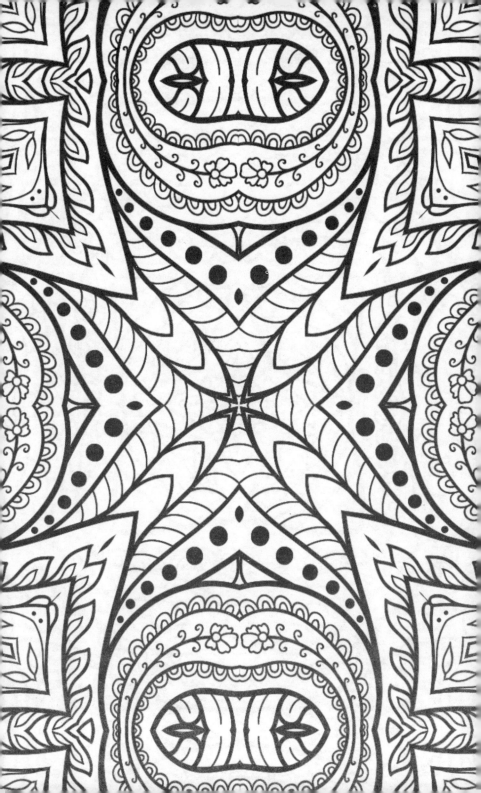

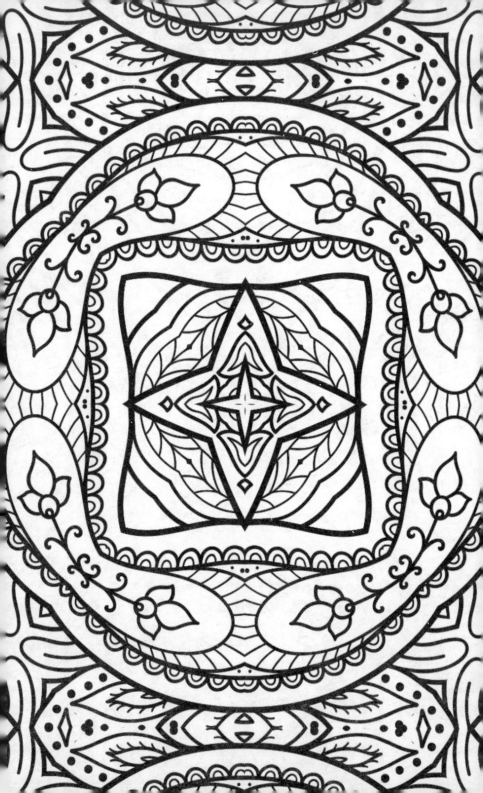

8. BIG BELLY LAUGH

When I was a kid, I got in trouble all the time for laughing at inappropriate times. I laughed when people got hurt, not because it was funny but because I was so freaked out all I could do was laugh. My mom made me write out, *"I will not laugh when people get hurt."* Hundreds of lines. There is research to support that laughter is the best medicine. And when it comes to burnout recovery, big belly laughs are healthy.

You can't fake this one. This isn't laughing at your spouse's bad jokes. This is a deep, belly laugh, a you're about to pee your pants laugh. Maybe a you actually do pee your pants laugh. You snort laugh. Or a soda comes out of your nose laugh.

You get the picture.

This one is so good! A big, deep, belly laugh stimulates your diaphragm. And guess what that stimulates? YES... your vagus nerve.

List your top 10 favorite movies you can turn to for a great big belly laugh!

1. _____   6. _____

2. _____   7. _____

3. _____   8. _____

4. _____   9. _____

5. _____   10. _____

9. NATURE

When I was in recovery, I walked around a lake. I loved a certain bench because it was in between a bunch of great big trees. I'd imagine roots coming out of my feet and sunshine coming down through the top of my head, kissing every cell of my body. Being out in nature without my phone helped me relax in massive ways. I'd automatically sigh, yawn, laugh, and experience release after release. Sometimes, I'd have big ugly cries, too.

Hanging out in nature reduces cortisol and helps you get present. You'll relax and probably sigh! Walking around your neighborhood is a great way to start, and be sure to keep your phone in your pocket or at home altogether. Take this one a bit further, though, and go hang out by a tree, or take a buddy and go for a walk on the beach, through the woods, or around a preserve.

Check out your neighborhood, community, and state for hiking/walking trails, awesome trees and green parks, lakes, creeks, and even sandy beaches. Make a list of your favorite spots you've already tried and know are safe and well populated. Then find a new nature spot you can go visit. Be sure to check out reviews and take a buddy!

Favorite trails:

_____

Favorite parks:

_____

Favorite trees:

_____

New nature spots to check out:

_____

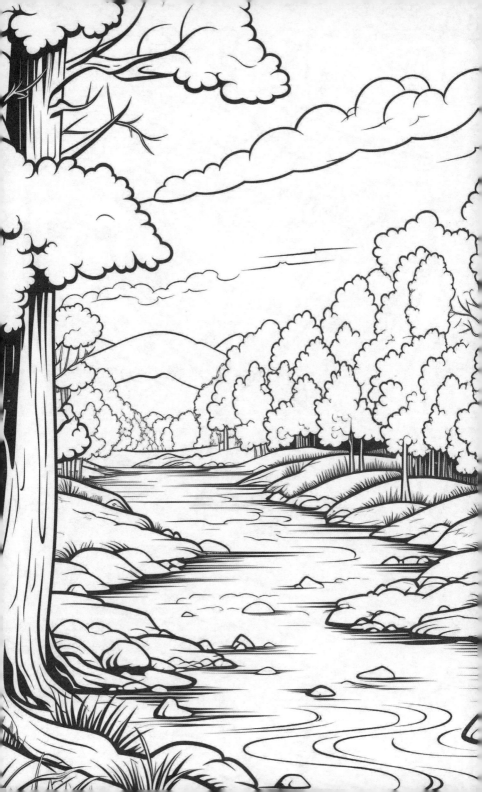

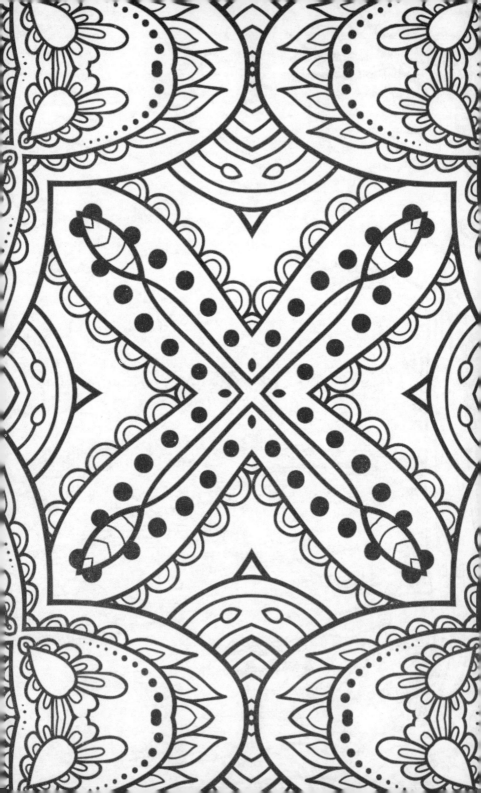

10. YAWNING

I force myself to yawn when I'm overly stressed. When I'm working on a big project and I can feel myself getting anxious, I will check out a video of someone yawning just to get me to yawn!

  Yawning stimulates the vagus nerve. Again with the vagus nerve, right? I'm telling you— it works! I bet you just yawned. Did you yawn? You did, right? Email me if I'm right.

How does your body feel after yawning?

_____

_____

_____

_____

_____

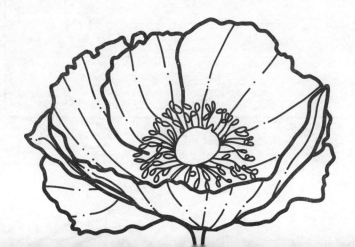

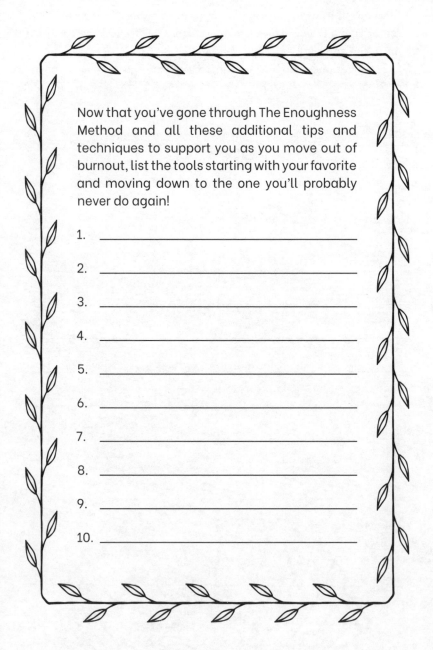

Now that you've gone through The Enoughness Method and all these additional tips and techniques to support you as you move out of burnout, list the tools starting with your favorite and moving down to the one you'll probably never do again!

1. _____

2. _____

3. _____

4. _____

5. _____

6. _____

7. _____

8. _____

9. _____

10. _____

Reclaiming your power, worth, and peace after burnout is as real as burnout itself. The road to recovery after burnout has not been a straightforward one for me. I slipped up several times, landing back in a state of being overwhelmed more times than I care to admit.

The workaholic in me is as real as the empathic one and the intuitive one. I love all the pieces within me the same. With time and experience came acceptance. Burnout is a darkness I learned to call my friend because it is within me. After a decade of experiencing it for the first time, I know when I'm heading toward it again.

When I'm working through lunches, taking calls during my scheduled breaks, and not putting energy into my self-care, I know burnout is next.

It happens every single time.

So, let's make a pact—okay, friend?

Promise me you'll take care of yourself. I'll promise you I'll take care of myself. And we'll share these tools with others so we all heal ourselves.

I love you.

Unapologetically.

xo,

Carrie

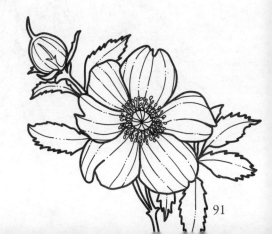

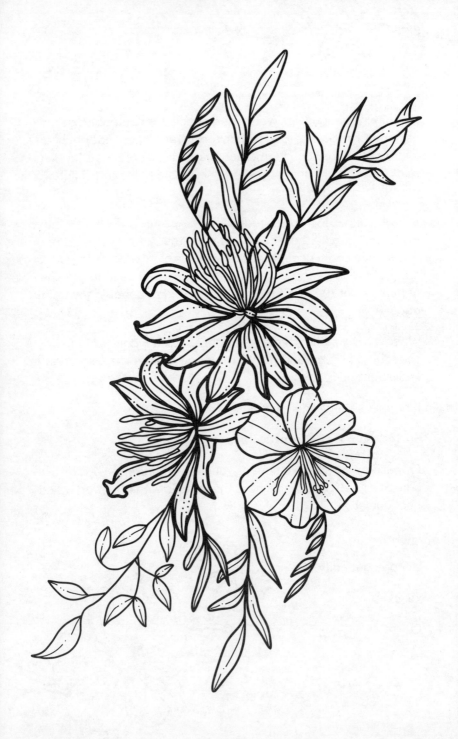

APPENDIX

CHECKLIST OF 10 BURNOUT RECOVERY TECHNIQUES

- ☐ Meditation
- ☐ Havening
- ☐ 4-7-8
- ☐ Tapping
- ☐ Humming
- ☐ Singing
- ☐ Sighing
- ☐ Yawning
- ☐ Laughing
- ☐ Nature

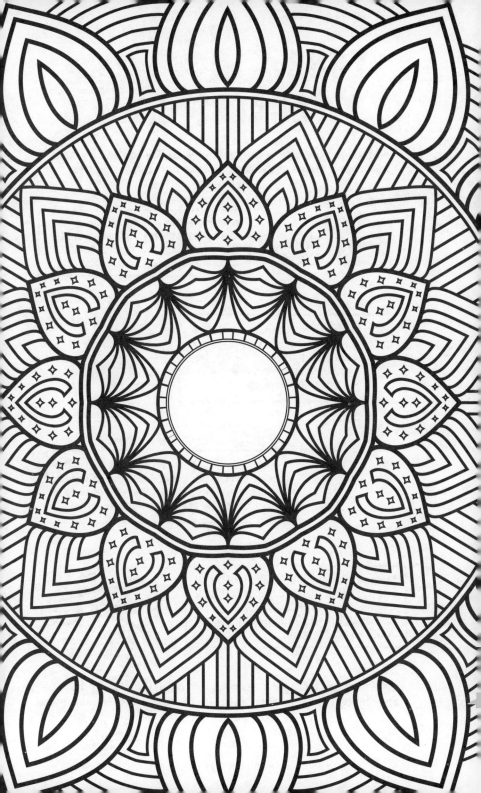

YOUR *Enoughness* ACCESSORY

Manage your stress throughout your day to keep burnout away! These self-care tips take only a few minutes.

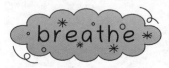

Increase focus and *mindfulness* while *decreasing stress*. Exhale 4 counts. Hold your breath 4 counts. Inhale 4 counts. Exhale 4 counts. Repeat!

Sit in the grass for 10-minutes. Notice the colors, smells, sounds, feelings and even tastes. And if there's a nearby tree, go hug it and exhale! 🌳
Nature is healing!

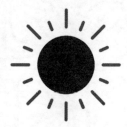

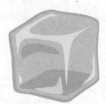

Grab something frozen and place it on the side of your neck for 60-seconds. Change sides and hold for another 60-seconds. Exhale. *This is my personal favorite!*

Engage your diaphragm and belt out... Happy Birthday to you! Happy Birthday to you! Happy Birthday, *DEAR YOOOUUUU...* 🎶 🎵 Happy Birthday to you! Repeat 3 times!

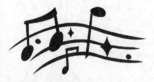

Remember this throughout your day... You are ENOUGH and you can move through stressful situations with the right tools. Practice these. Love yourself. XOXO
Carrie

I AM
enough

I AM
resourceful

I AM
amazing

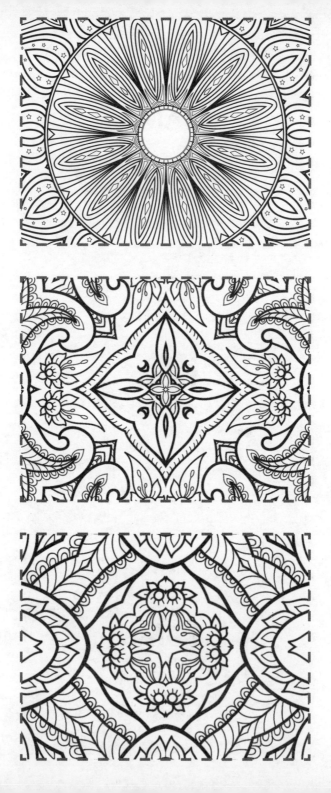

I AM
capable

I AM
recovering from burnout

I AM
loving to myself

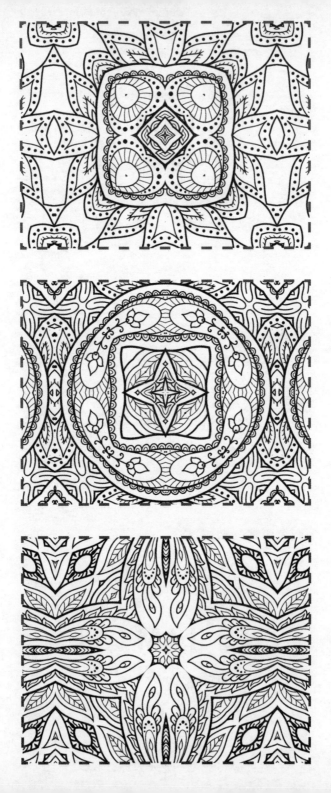

I AM

my own best friend

I AM

positively changing my life

I AM

proud of myself

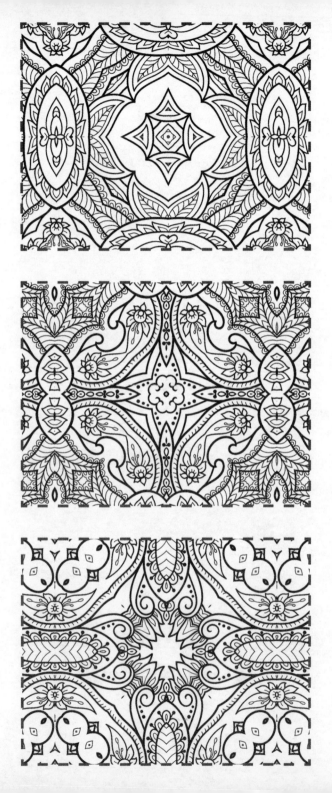

I AM

_____

I AM

_____

I AM

_____

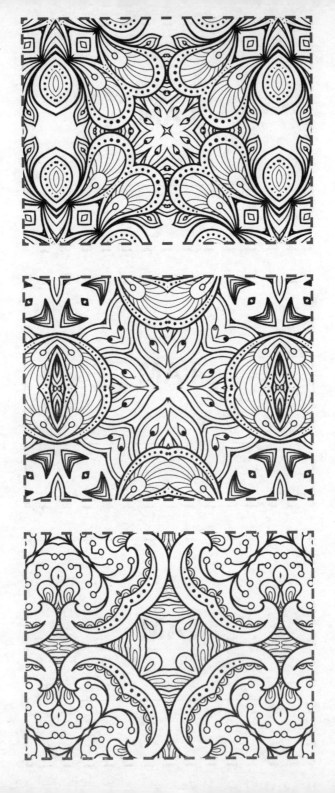

I AM

_____

I AM

_____

I AM

_____

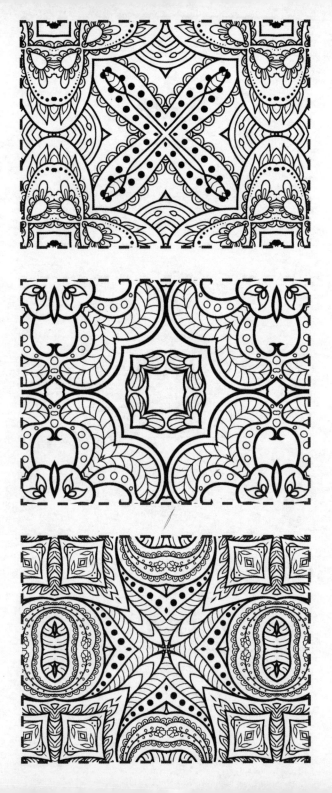

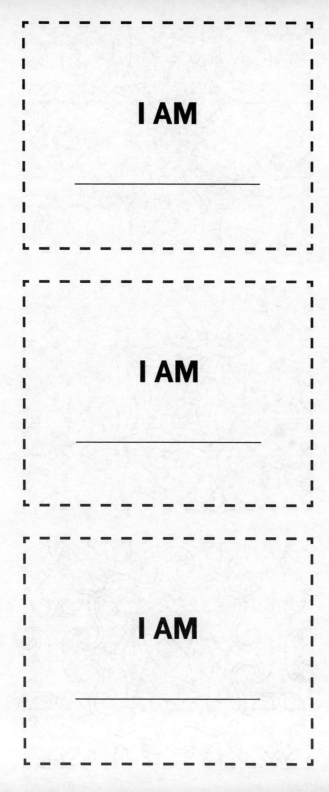

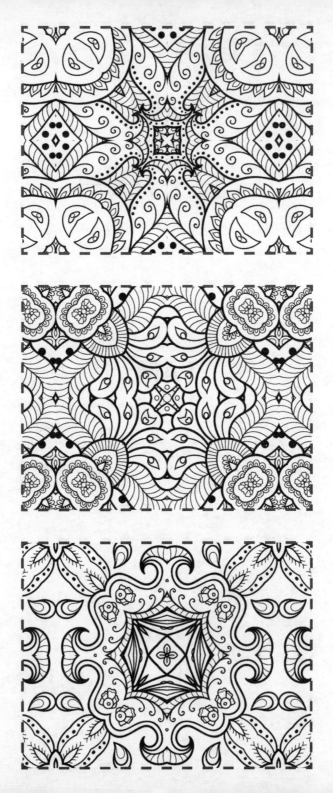

I AM

_____

I AM

_____

I AM

_____

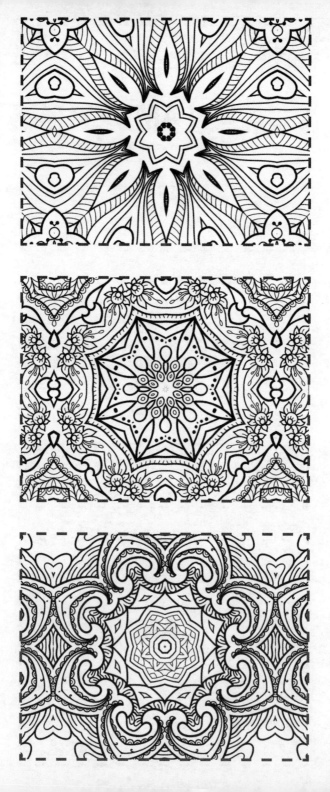

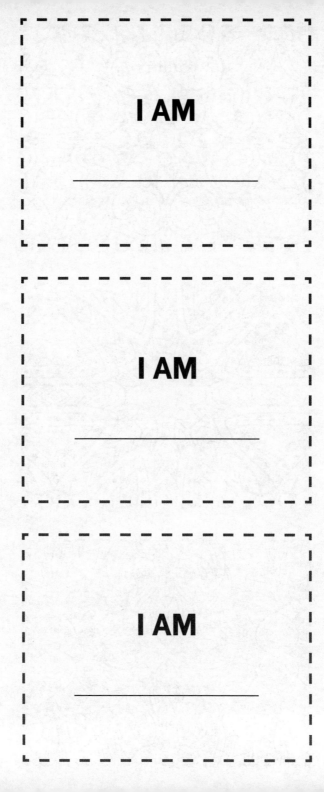

I AM

_____

I AM

_____

I AM

_____

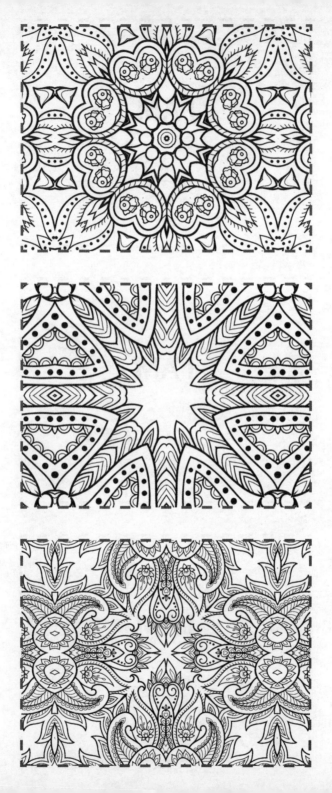

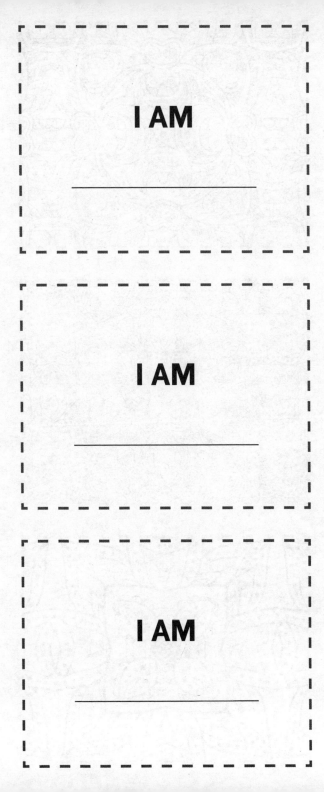

I AM

———————————

I AM

———————————

I AM

———————————

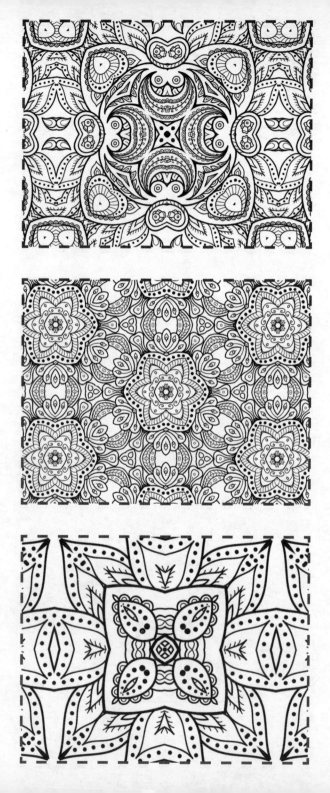

Acknowledgments

Normally, authors use this space to acknowledge all the people who supported them in the journey to create their book. The people who support me in my work as an author know how much I love them and how grateful I am for each and every one of them.

Phone calls always end with, "I love you." We hug all the time. Text, phone, and emails galore.

My heartfelt acknowledgment and appreciation is to the readers who are in burnout and praying this helps them move through it and come out of it.

I pray that for you, too.

The Enoughness Method came about first because I was burned out and had to find a way out. The idea to put this little book together was the result of a solid year of working with healthcare professionals who were in burnout.

What I told all of them was this: Burnout is the result of unmanaged, prolonged stress. It won't go away after a long weekend or a vacation. You have to create new pathways for yourself and your nervous system. If you do that, things will change.

I love you.

You've got this.

About the Author

CARRIE SEVERSON is the author of *The Enoughness Method &
Unapologetically Enough*. She delivers burnout recovery talks and workshops to audiences both large and small. She is married, living in Arizona,
and currently working on her next book about walking alongside her husband, Gavin, through his cancer journey.

**Connect with her on her social media platforms or at
www.CarrieSeverson.com.**

Facebook.com/carrieseverson.storyteller
Instagram.com/the_unapologetic_voice_house
Tiktok.com/@carrieseverson